The Art
of
Mental Wellbeing

The Polarity of Mental Wellbeing
& Mental Disorder Beyond the
Medical Approach

The Art of Mental Wellbeing
The Polarity of Mental Wellbeing & Mental Disorder
Beyond the Medical Approach

Published in Great Britain 2003 by

MASTERWORKS INTERNATIONAL
27 Old Gloucester Street
London
WC1N 3XX
England

Tel: 0780 3173272
Email: books@masterworksinternational.com
Web: http://www.masterworksinternational.com

The Art of Mental Wellbeing

The Polarity of Mental Wellbeing & Mental Disorder
Beyond the Medical Approach

By Tony Caves

Contents

Acknowledgements

It is said that all originality is undiscovered plagiarism so this work is dedicated to everyone I have ever spoken to and every book I have ever read!

Any merit in this work is entirely due to my Inner Teacher. All the errors are mine alone.

Wellbeing

"Health is a state of complete physical, mental and social wellbeing and not merely the absence of disease or infirmity"

World Health Organisation

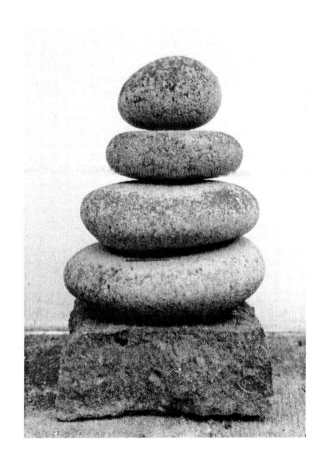

'Qi to the Power of Five'
A photograph by Rita Caves

INTRODUCTION

Setting the Scene

This book had its beginning in a very pertinent question asked many years ago by a training course participant who was an unqualified care assistant in a 'home' for mentally disordered people. She said, "OK, the doctor has been and prescribed the pills or injection and has now gone. What can we on the sharp end of the caring process do now—bearing in mind that the person now has the side effects of the drugs to cope with as well as the symptoms." This whole work is an attempt to answer that question.

This is a real and enduring difficulty. For generations in this and other countries people have waited until they became ill and then consulted medical practitioners expecting a cure, usually in the form of a lotion or potion, or in more extreme cases surgical intervention. These procedures were supposed to make them well and their own involvement in this process is minimal, as if the answer to our healing is somehow outside ourselves. This is the position today in the case of mental disorder.

We must begin to understand that there can be no cure or wellbeing without effort on the part of the person suffering from the disorder. There is no magic solution. No panacea that will put it all right. The disordered persons themselves must be involved in becoming well, must be committed to it personally. The healing resonance must be present in the individual. The methods can then be very simple but very powerful, working at the level of energy, vitality, *vervality* and resonance. In this way we are working beyond the coarse do it by numbers medical approach.

What I have sought to discover over the years are methods with which an individual can work themselves out of disorder. Methods that work below the level of symptom and will be effective in spite of the drugs. This will mean the individual being empowered to make informed decisions about treatment. Working on the basis that we are all the same, but we are all different, it will include valuing difference and change. Changing behaviour allows feeling to follow. Changing thinking allows both behaviour and feelings to follow. Practising activities which bring about these changes increases resonance toward a healthy transparency in our lives.

Transparency is an everyday state of awareness that enables us to feel centred and clear about who and where we are. We feel ok about not being in control, ok about the fuzzy edges of reality and constant change. We are content to work with the flow and process of life in the here and now. However, the most important point I can make, is that we must be aware that transparency is not a goal, it is not the destination of perfection that when we arrive we have somehow 'made it'.

We must remember we are just passing through on our way from birth to death. This body, brain and personality are just things we use on the way to experience many shades of joy and sorrow. They are not permanent, each one changing from moment to moment. Within this situation nothing stands by itself, there is no independent existence. We are all dependent upon one another.

Tony Caves Brighton 2003

Because the eye looks
but can catch no glimpse of it,
it is called elusive.

Because the ear listens
but cannot hear it,
it is called rarefied.

Because the hand feels for it
but cannot touch it,
it is called, infinitesimal.

Its rising brings no light
Its setting no darkness
It is called Qi.

Tao Te Ching

PROLOGUE

The Hypothesis

"Great spirits are always opposed by mediocre minds." Albert Einstein.

This book arose from my practice working with mentally disordered people and designing and teaching courses and workshops for staff, carers and survivors of service. It has been my experience that mental disorder is born from pain and fear that lead to the expression of negative feelings and emotions. It has also been my observation that we are not finite 'things' – solid, separate, permanent, continuous and defined (as Ngakchang Rinpoche puts it), that can be 'treated,' but a series of energetic processes ever changing and eminently changeable. It appears to me that mental disorder or 'illness' begins as a functional disorder and develops over quite long periods of time, into an organic one in which the body/brain system begins to deteriorate thus masking the causes. However, this is reversible at any stage, not by treating the physical symptoms, but the underlying functional causes.

That is the hypothesis here, that mental disorder can be worked with, not at the level of symptom, but at the level of cause. This work can only be done by the person with the disorder—the most we can do is assist by providing an explanation of what is happening, a structure for the work to take place and a series of techniques.

In respect of mental wellbeing and mental disorder the prevailing orthodoxy is psychiatry. The problem with orthodoxy is that it always attempts to increase power and oppose change. Within the orthodoxy no dissent is allowed.

Those who seriously challenge the system are vilified. As examples, Peter Breggin in America is a virtual outcast of the psychiatric community and Scottish psychiatrist R.D. Laing was eventually struck off the medical register. These systems are a circular dead-end where the entrance is also the exit. Like all 'professions' orthodoxy's are a refuge for the mediocre with an incredibly impoverished view of the world.

The study of mental disorder is not enough to bring about sanity. In fact the study of mental disorder actually creates madness. It is my experience that psychiatry has spectacularly failed to find any answers to the problem of mental disorder. At its best psychiatry subdues symptoms and allows a low level of functioning absent of any form of creativity. At its worst, through diagnosis or labelling, psychiatry creates mentally-ill people who become long term habitual prescribed drug takers, presenting all the symptoms of their particular 'mental illness' for the rest of their lives. It is my opinion that, underwritten by the 'Big Pharma' – the international legalised drugs racket – high salary psychiatrists and psychologists are usually involved in profitable, selective, repeat business. Thus we should remove mental disorder from a medical context. However, for the moment it seems to be all that is on offer as a response to mental disorder.

A second part to the hypotheses is to do with what some people have called 'life energy' – what the Chinese philosophers and practitioners called 'Qi' (pron. Chee). Interestingly, modern astronomers and physicists, realizing that space is not a vacuum, used a similar word 'quintessence' to describe the basic 'field of the universe.' I believe that 'Qi-sense' is a useful word to use in this context to describe this phenomenon because it bridges the gap between ancient and modern thinking. Most descriptions I have read about 'life energy' make it sound linear and flat—energy or power that although vibrational in nature can be made to move in one direction and is ordered to the point of ossification. However, what I call 'Qi-sense' is a non linear. constantly moving, undulating and changing frequency of electro-magnetic resonance. It does not need wires and has its own self organising integrity. However, it is susceptible to resistance and is expressed in degrees of density. In the human body a resistance occurs at the skin of the individual and usually only the most subtle Qi-sense passes through this resistance. Different densities occur from sparkling electrical phenomena to the congealed Qi-sense of the physical world. In order to experience Qi-sense in ourselves and the world, practice at experiencing this skin barrier resistance and softening the congealed nature of Qi-sense expressed as physicality is required. These practices lead to what some people describe as having 'an incredible lightness of being' and is what I term transparency. In terms of working with Qi-sense, positive or negative energy is the same thing and the name of the game is transformation. That is the major theme of this book.

I first became aware of Qi-sense as a young martial arts student learning Judo and Karate. One of the very senior Japanese instructors told me to stand facing him some three metres away. He then performed a slow sweeping 'air punch' with the open palm of his hand moving toward me. I was waiting for him to rush forward and attack, but he stayed where he was. Much to my surprise I felt a wave of 'something' pass through me that made me bend forward and feel slightly sick. A usually stern man he smiled at me and waggled his finger playfully. It was a pity he could not speak English because I was hooked and wanted to know what this phenomenon was. Since then I have become more aware that it is the very basis of all we are and the world we inhabit. It manifests in different frequencies and densities and can be used to harm and heal. The importance of that initial demonstration was that it showed that this electro-magnetic resonance or Qi-sense can be experienced, worked with and transmitted from one individual to another.

A third part to the hypotheses is concerned with empowerment and valuing difference. As humans we are all very much the same in the way we look and think, our bodies tend to have two arms two legs and a head. Myths from different parts of the world reflect remarkably similar themes. Yet we are vastly different in our interpretation and expression, we move very differently and express our similar ideas in a vast array of different ways. We reflect infinite diversity in infinite combinations while remaining essentially the same. This is the paradoxical nature of our existence as a human family.

In ancient times initiates of the hidden mysteries referred to themselves as 'cosmopolitan.' They felt that their initiation experience transcended nationalistic, ethnic and religious boundaries and closed thinking and that they were citizens of the world. They had been 'empowered' in the true sense of the word. Following their lead we can say that Qi-sense is not just an eastern, Chinese or Japanese experience but a human one.

It is interesting that there are no precise words in English to describe what I call Qi-sense This means that people whose only language is English have no access to the concept and this puts them at a distinct disadvantage – 'life energy' being a very poor description. The Eskimo have many words for snow. The Chinese Taoist and Buddhist philosophers have many words for Qi-sense. The main one as we have already discussed is 'Qi.' This is the very basic stuff which is the resonance of the whole universe. There are versions of Qi called Jing and Shen. The definitions of these words are often difficult and abstruse. However, it is perhaps helpful in relation to connectedness and unconnectedness to think of Qi as all encompassing mind essence, Jing as specifically associated with the body/brain complex and Shen as the stuff of conscious awareness, that identifies us as sentient beings. When there is a free flow of Qi, Jing and Shen individuals live their lives at peak capacity, they are alert but grounded, everything seems to 'click' and they are fully engaged with the flow of events. We must remember that power and energy are very poor descriptions of this phenomena that underlies our lives. It is more useful to think of Qi, Jing and Shen as verbs rather than nouns. When they vibrate clearly within our lives we feel transparent. In this book, I will use the word Qi-sense to describe the electro-magnetic resonance that leads to clarity and transparency. We need to adopt or access an English lexicon to raise awareness and understanding of something as important to humanity as snow is to the Eskimo.

Although very subtle and hard to define, Qi-sense underlies everything in the universe. It fills the 'void' of space and congealed it becomes matter. Within our world it is visible in five ways. It is in the solidity of the earth, the fluidity of water, the combustion of fire, the motility of air and the primal energy of space. Humans appreciate it through the use of the five senses sight (light), hearing (sound), touch (kinaesthetic), smell (breathing), and taste (eating). We work with these five senses in three ways through thinking, action and feeling.

We are very fortunate to write speak and understand contemporary English for this is a truly cosmopolitan language. It is full of words that have their origin in virtually every other language of the world and more are added every day, it is constantly in transition. That is the value of English, we can adopt and use words that explain things that are beyond the scope of more limited linguistics.

This why there is no problem adopting, valuing and practising ideas from anywhere in the world. In this book you will find ideas and practices from China to ancient Greece, Africa to Australia and even the new age; in fact anything that provides an authentic, universally valid, human experience leading to clarity and transparency.

17

Clear understanding of our Qi-sense, being, behaviour and thinking processes does exist. It is encoded in systems such as Tibetan Buddhism and Neuro-linguistic programming – Polarity Therapy, Meditation, Tai-Ji and Qi-Gong. The ordinary Buddhist practitioner has more understanding of the nature of mind than most of our eminent professionals. There are centres of excellence and change. But these are few and far between. As always change is brought about by fringe and voluntary bodies and organisations, survivors groups and a few brave individuals. I hope this book may in some small, quiet, non-sectarian way contribute to this movement.

Existence is a puzzle of constantly
Interchanging pieces
Our error is in seeing the puzzle as
The ultimate riddle to be solved
For in reflecting on the solution
We blind ourselves to the reality that
When all the pieces are in place
There is no puzzle.

Anon

CHAPTER 1

Polarity, Triunity, Cinquinicity

"All things accord in number."   Pythagoras

It may seem odd to begin a book about mental well being discussing number. However, proportion and metaphor are powerful tools in thinking about this particular topic. Rationality is fine in the world of the intellect. However, when the intellect is impaired by disorder, rational solutions become increasingly useless. We find that life consists of infinite diversity in infinite variations, constantly in motion. The rigid 'scientific' world of 2+2=4 is a world of conceptual abstraction and when we attempt to apply this model to real life experience we invariably meet the fuzzy, rough edges of reality. This is a practical book for people who 'DO' and people who experience disorder. In these instances other ideas, explanations and methods are needed to enable the person to work themselves toward wellbeing. Taking numbers that appear to have meaning and which structure our world and using them as metaphors to give meaning to our existence is a very powerful and empowering thing to do.

The Pythagoreans, an ancient group of practical mystic philosophers whose order survives to this day, hold that everything is number and the explanation and workings of the whole universe is contained in the numbers 1-10 or 0-9 both of which give us ten digits. The Pythagoreans constructed ten as a triangular number as follows: 1+2+3+4=10, which they termed the Holy Decad. Hence the saying among them that 'four is ten' and their symbol the Tetraktys (fig.1). In terms of thought and human interaction with the world and with each other they hold that the most important numbers within the Holy Decad are two, three and five. In the mystery teachings of ancient times these numbers were known as the 'three sacred roots' and were intrinsically linked with the teaching of the Vesica piscis (fig.1), a misunderstanding, or maybe knowledge, of which led the Christians to adopt the fish as their symbol.

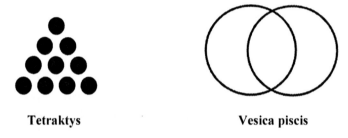

Tetraktys **Vesica piscis**

Fig. 1

As a very simple outline of this knowledge, the square roots of two, three and five are all the root relationships necessary for the formation of the five regular Platonic solids. These are also the only numbers required to divide the octave into musical scales. Called 'The Law of Three' in geometric demonstration these 'irrational roots' are the generators of pure archetypal processes from which emerge whole, fixed numbers which provide structure and content. Transformation is thus a process of generation (2), formation (3), and regeneration (5), or energy, matter, flux. This process is at the heart of work with disorder and wellbeing because the blocking of this process of transformation means stagnation and sickness.

Polarity

So what does this all mean in practical terms? Life springs from duality in a process of generation. We live day to day in a dualistic world, opposites are the very foundation of our experience here in this place we call the universe, left/right, light/dark, right/wrong. In terms of the polarity of mental wellbeing and mental disorder it is essential to understand the nature and function of duality.

The Pythagoreans called this the *'apeiron pneuma kosmoi'* – the great breath of the universe. They taught that the universe alternately expands and contracts over aeons of time. This is a circular process with no beginning and no end. At this point in time we are in a process of expansion, so the 'big bang' theory is half right. This circular centrifugal/ centripetal action is true of everything in the universe including ourselves. Sometime before our birth our Qi-sense begins to expand, it goes through the birth experience and into life. At some point, different for everyone, it begins to contract, pass through the death experience and into the interlife period to a point where expansion starts again and proceeds to birth. This goes on endlessly and is what some Buddhists call Samsara, a cycle they seek to escape by achieving the non-duality of enlightenment.

Across the millennia there have been many attempts to describe this dualistic principle using different approaches and imagery, sun and moon, fire and ice, wisdom and compassion, anima and animus, it is the snowflake in the storm of fire. Perhaps, however, the most comprehensive explanation comes again from Chinese Taoist and Buddhist thinkers and practitioners who spoke of two principles they called yin and yang – again words which may be familiar to English readers and are encapsulated in the Tai-Ji; the supreme ultimate symbol of the universe (fig.2). These are the two basic conditions that spring from Qi and everything in the universe is made up of a flexing resulting from their interaction; each contains the seed of its opposite in an endless relationship of interplay and harmony.

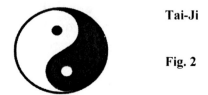

Tai-Ji

Fig. 2

Yin is the female receptive side of our nature. This is the creative force that gives us the reasons for our actions, forming our insights into new ideas and thinking. This is the capacity to assimilate new values, beliefs and concepts. It provides our creative energies, our appreciation of beauty and our sense of wonder. It often shows in our daydreams or at night when we are sleeping. It allows our minds to go free, to float and drift and encourages lateral modes of thinking. It enables us to nurture, support and care for ourselves and others. In our society it is often marginalized, distorted and devalued. Not being in touch with this wisdom aspect of our nature can lead to mental disorder.

Yang is the masculine active side of our nature. This is our physical energetic self that gives us the drive and energy needed to carry out our tasks and ideas, dreams and desires. It enables us to think in logical, concrete and structured ways and is our outward expression. It enables us to protect, defend and provide for ourselves and others. In our society this aspect is over emphasised and people not behaving successfully in these ways are seen as failing or non-productive. The over emphasis of power and dominance characteristic of this part of our nature can lead people toward mental disorder. When yang is viewed as active compassion it leads to transparency.

Yin and Yang characterize the endless interplay of

opposites that compliment and change one another in an endless spiral dance. However, at some time during the development of our Eurocentric culture, polarity and duality came to mean something very different from the prevailing world view. The advent of 'rationality' brought the notion of the universe in conflict. The battle between the abstract and the concrete, the ideal and the real. Things became either one thing or another and there is a sharp divide based on binary logic and evidential truth! This mind versus matter attitude gave rise to the authoritarian viewpoint that dominates mainstream work with mentally disordered people to this day. This is the authoritarian notion of what Kramer and Alstad call the 'goodself' and the 'badself.'

The authoritarian idea of the goodself and the badself is at the very root of the accepted medically based 'treatment' of mental disorder. In this system we cannot trust ourselves and need an external authority figure to whom we surrender to make us 'good' and psychotropic drugs to keep us in that position.

The view of duality that allows that we are sometimes up and sometimes down and sometimes in-between and an awareness that this is subject to constant change leads to our being well in ourselves. Being comfortable in one's own skin and not attempting to constantly get to that unattainable state of goodness. Empowerment stresses and promotes self trust because without self trust and occasional mistakes we cannot move toward growth and wholeness. In all times and in all places we always have choices and these are largely a matter of perception. We must learn to trust ourselves to make the best possible choice based on our perception of the situation. Enabling this is empowerment.

The limitations of the either/or position are illustrated by the old question of whether a river is the water or the banks it flows through. The answer must be both because neither would be river without the other.

Triunity

Triunity is duality with what some writers have termed 'the resolving third' that brings about formation. By becoming 'tri' it achieves 'unity' moving to a both/and analogue position. All dualistic constructions call for this resolving third that is paradoxically the same but separate from the seeming opposites and acts as a catalyst. It is not balance but tends like life and nature toward a temporary but constantly moving equilibrium. It is the root of the useful conceptual abstraction of past, present and future that we call time. We have clocks that measure time as a constant. But it is clear that we as humans do not always view time in this way. We have trite sayings that emphasise this, 'time flies when you're having fun' and 'the longest day.' Time is a flexible concept as is our most cherished notion that we have a separate, permanent identity. The good news is, from the point of view of mental disorder, it means our identity, personality, and behaviour are eminently changeable and thus 'reprogrammable.'

Three represents completeness; beginning, middle and end. It is present in all complete notions; three wishes, bronze, silver and gold, three wise men, three musketeers. It represents the three types of therapeutic touch used in Polarity Therapy[1]; satvic, tamasic, rajasic and the three energy vortices in the body, top of the head, golden section (just below the navel) and the bubbling spring on the soles of each foot. Three is a piercing of the binary, dualistic, polarity. It is a breaking through, going beyond the opposites to show the way to infinite potentiality. In the words of the Heart Sutra, 'Gate, Gate, Paragate' or as the auctioneer would say "Going, Going, Gone." This presence of '*throughness*' taking us past duality and making a new whole is the essence of wellbeing and transparency. People who are mentally disordered have

26

limited their options to the closed duality of this or that and view everything in life from the viewpoint of disorder and perplexity. Three shows that at any point in our lives there are endless possibilities open to each individual.

Three is the only number in the Decad to equal the sum of all the other terms below it; 3=2+1. It is also the only number whose sum with those below it equals their product; 1+2+3=1x2x3. In this way it reflects the Buddhist Dzogchen view that Samsara or dualistic conditioning, 1 and 2, is included in the notion of Nirvana which equals 3. Nirvana and Samsara are not separate or opposite, Nirvana equals the sum of all the terms below it and the sum with those below it equals the product—Enlightenment.

As Pythagoras appeared to hint, becoming aware of tripartite patterns in our world will awaken our understanding of the true nature of our existence within that world and of the nature of thought as brain, mind and conscious awareness.

Cinquinicity

Cinquinicity describes the essence and form of the number five in all its manifestations. Five is an incredible number, halfway between one and ten, it is the number of regeneration and therefore healing, especially self healing. Five perfects and completes everything within the duality and triunity. The ancient Egyptians saw it as the number of illumination. Five is the basis of the practical applications of the specific techniques chapter of this book.

The square root of five gives us phi or the golden section or mean, that the Pythagoreans called the divine proportion. It is found in everything from the length of our bones to the way leaves grow on a plant. The golden section derives from the Vesica piscis, and shows the relationship of equivalency between two ratios and is the reason the ancient Christians used the fish as their symbol copying the initiates of the mystery traditions. The golden section can be explained thus; the smaller term is to the larger as the whole is to the larger plus the smaller. Until recent times this was considered a great secret. All classical Greek temples are built to the phi proportion and in ancient times it was concealed in the Old Testament which was a reworking of even older texts. 'In the beginning was the word and the word was with God and the word was God' or a is to b as b is to (a+b). Word is to God as God is to (Word + God).

Five is found everywhere in nature and in our constructed world. The Fibonacci numbers show that phi is present in the spacing of seeds in a sunflower, natural spirals like that of a snail shell, in the distribution of leaves on a plant and in the formation of crystalline structures. The ratios of the human form accord to phi and in the height of the body it occurs at what Daoist practitioners call the Dantian, two inches below the navel and back towards the centre of the torso. The very point of balance. We have five fingers on each hand, five toes on each foot and five major internal organs heart, lungs, liver, kidneys and spleen.

The archetypal representation of pentagonal symmetry is the five-pointed star or pentagram (fig.3). Look around, it appears everywhere and has a deep psychological significance for people all over the world. The heroes of our society become 'superstars' and it appears on the flags of many nations as well as a host of corporate logos worldwide.

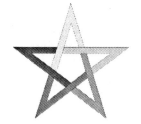

The Five Pointed Star
or
Pentagram

Fig. 3

Properly constructed the five-pointed star contains ten golden sections and echoes other sets of ten close to us like ten fingers and ten toes. Join the points of the star and we have the pentagon, the name and shape of the military headquarters of the most powerful nation on earth. Two plus ten pentagons, gives us the dodecahedron which is one of the five Platonic solids.

Cinquinicity is most effectively portrayed in the Egyptian pyramid. The four corners at the base of the pyramid represent the four 'base' elements earth, air, fire and water. The point at the apex represents the elusive fifth element known to the Alchemists as 'quintessence' which represents the Qi-sense nature of the universe and is the medium or plenum within which the other four elements function. The five faces of the pyramid also represent the five elements in inverse proportion. The upper faces representing the four 'base' elements with the face on the ground the fifth element – 'as above, so below'. Within the Great Pyramid there are also five 'relieving chambers' that have recently been associated with acoustic effects. It has been said that they amplified the extra low frequency of the resonant field (sometimes called the Schumann resonance), of the planet, so that it became audible as a low rumble across the Giza Plateau. Perhaps they also gave the vibrational frequencies of the five elements that could be used by the priest and priestesses for healing.

The most ancient descriptions (as well as most modern ones) of Qi-sense within and around the body speak of five chakras, khorlos or wheels (fig.4) and five pathways of moving energy within and around the body flowing between our five fingers and toes (fig.5). It is the functioning or flexing of Qi-energy in both concert and free flow along organised pathways that leads to physical and mental well being. The wheels and pathways match the five elements in terms of sound colour and vibration.

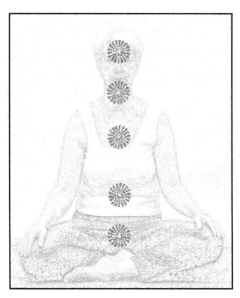

Positions of the five chakras,
khorlos or wheels of Qi-sense
Fig. 4

Working toward mental well being we access Qi-sense through the five senses that produce the five representational systems we use to build our inner and outer worlds. Thus we represent the world through the five inner and the five outer senses; visual, auditory, kinaesthetic, gustatory and olfactory. Mental disorder comes about through a perplexed appreciation of the world through these representational systems. The good news is that all thinking is open to a process of change and the premise of the techniques in this book is that we can work toward transparency and clarity of thinking, feeling and action.

Chakras

There are different ideas relating to the number of chakras in the human body. Different systems advocate five, seven or sometimes nine. These systems are all contained within the very ancient pre-dynastic 'Egyptian' teachings of the House of Life of 'Beloved Sekhmet' – the one who was before the gods were,' whose name means 'powerful one,' so named because the practices were concerned with the understanding and use of Qi-sense. The five chakra system was the basic set for used for healing physicality (body and brain). They understood the divine proportions within the human body that reflected the perplexity or transparency of Qi-sense.

The philosopher Pythagoras was an initiate of this very secret order, whose teachings have largely been lost, but the remnants of which are contained in the Pythagorean oral tradition. Very little is known about these priest and priestesses because they were outside the mainstream of Egyptian religious life. They recognised no external authority, admitted men and women on equal merit and had no hierarchy, as they all viewed themselves as an expression of 'Beloved Sekhmet,' whom they regarded as their 'inner

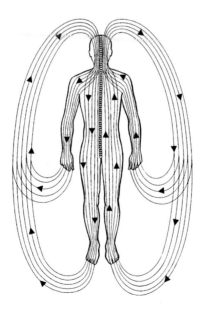

Fig 5   The Five Pathways of Qi-sense

31

teacher.' That is why there are no statues of the them , only of 'Beloved Sekhmet.'

The five chakras were worked in respect of physical (body/brain) healing. In terms of teachings about death two chakras were added, the red drop of Qi-sense, gained from the mother at conception, and the white drop, gained from the father at conception, that unite with the resolving third at the heart/mind at the moment of death. For advanced spiritual practice the heaven chakra above the head (positive energy pole) and earth chakra below the feet (negative energy pole) were indicated. These are shown on statues of 'Beloved Sekhmet' as the sun disc (that was later portrayed as a halo) and an oblong plinth beneath the feet. These positive and negative energies are the same as those worked within Polarity Therapy[1] and later became mistakenly portrayed as heaven and hell because they are drawn into the heart/mind with the drops at the point of death.

The spiritual practices of the priest and priestesses was a closely guarded secret and involved using the heaven and earth chakras through the whole chakra system to duplicate the process of the death experience at the level of the Qi-sense while remaining in life. This was known as the 'little death' and gave practitioners an ethereal but totally empowered quality that led to them being feared and shunned, although highly respected, by the rest of society. This gave rise to misconceived ideas about crucifixion and resurrection.

The practices outlined in this book would have been basic to their work.

---

1. Polarity Therapy is a form of energy based healing discovered by and taught by the polymath Dr Randolph Stone DC DO ND

Symbols of metaphor for wellbeing and transparence

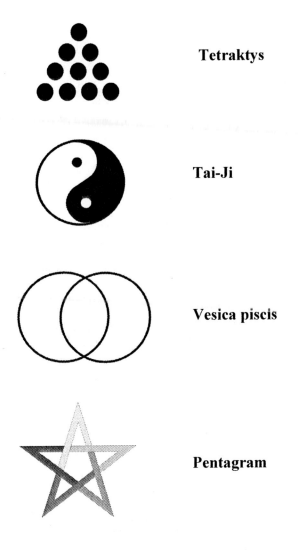

Tetraktys

Tai-Ji

Vesica piscis

Pentagram

Everything is energy in motion. A human being is a part of the whole, called by us 'universe', a part limited in time and space. He experiences himself, his thoughts and feelings as something separated from the rest—a kind of optical delusion of his consciousness.

This delusion is a kind of prison for us, restricting us to our personal desires and to affection for a few persons nearest to us.

Our task must be to free ourselves from this prison by widening our circle of compassion to embrace all living creatures and the whole of nature in its beauty.

Albert Einstein

CHAPTER 2

Brain, Mind & Consciousness

"Everything in the universe is composed of constantly changing energy."
Denise Linn

This chapter presents one way of looking at how we think and the process of thinking. It seeks to discover what constitutes 'disordered' thinking and what makes for 'healthy' thought processes and what it is that makes us who we are. It is a way that has proven helpful to me and to others and will hopefully prove helpful to the reader of this work. It is taken from ancient ideas and practices but firmly based in the authors' face to face research and practice with mentally disordered people, including the criminally insane, and those who work with them. It is a mixture of rationality and analogy for I do not believe, for instance, that Tibetan cosmology and scientific method are mutually exclusive, they are both valid within their own sphere. However, in any explanation we should keep in the forefront of our understanding that the map is not the territory, it is just one way of 'getting a handle' on things.

This is a huge and complex topic but polarity is a useful starting point inasmuch as basic brain thinking leads to a twofold appreciation – we are either attracted to the object of our thought or we feel aversion toward it, whatever 'it' may be and this distorts Qi-sense. This becomes triune through the addition of the resolving third – indifference and finding the energetic balance leads to free flow and clarity. Thus all our thinking is based in attraction (positive), aversion (negative) or indifference (neutral), which act with distortion or clarity within the cinquinicity of the five elements. In Polarity Therapy practice this equates to rajasic touch as stimulating, positive, forming – satvic contacts as balancing, neutral, energetic and tamasic touch as dispersing, negative, empty.

The structure of the thinking process can also be viewed as triune in nature. My research would lead me to the view that there are three aspects to the process and content of thinking and thought. These are; brain activity, consciousness and mind. We must continue to be aware, however, that these divisions are only there to help us get to grips with the topic – there is no real division. In the words of the Heart Sutra 'emptiness is form and form is emptiness.'

In terms of mental health and disorder, one only has to look at a corpse to see that the body and the brain which is part of the body, cannot become ill, sick or disordered by itself. An energising principle must be present to bring about changes. Without the energising principle it simply rots. Thus we have the physical organ of the brain which functions through a crude chemical/electrical mechanism and it is this mechanism that is the primary province of psychiatry and neurology and really where these disciplines stop. The drug therapy, electric shock treatment and surgical intervention of the "cut'em, shock'em and drug'em, brigade" all seek to intervene within this physical chemical and electrical system. These interventions appear not work, they merely subdue symptoms and replace them with the side effects of treatment, rather than restore full health.

There is a great deal of research at the moment, using mild electrical stimulus, to examine which areas of the brain are responsible for what thoughts. However, even this research is leading to the conclusion that many different areas of the brain are fired for each thought. Each time a thought takes place there is a consensus of lots of different pieces of information. The areas of the brain fired for the same thought might be different in different people. So, although the outcome may appear ordered the process is actually chaotic.

There are, however, documented accounts of people living 'normal lives,' even showing a good intelligence, with little or no physical brain at all and only fluid in the brain cavity. There is no evidence, however, of anyone living without a heart! Again, there are examples of extreme trauma to the head and brain, like spikes entering the lower back of the head and emerging through the bridge of the nose, having little or no effect on the individual once the initial difficulty has been stabilised. We must be aware that the thinking involved at the heart/mind level is not at the same density as the physical body/brain to which it steps down.

There is a movement on the fringes of scientific research which comes to the conclusion that to explain complex scientific ideas scientists must use the tools of poetry and metaphor because current scientific methodologies are wholly inadequate. It is also thought that our explanations and understanding of what happens actually influences events. So by and large what we expect to happen in any given set of circumstances is usually what will happen as long as enough of us believe it. In this way 'reality' is a consensus reflection of non-physical Qi-sense. When not observed every potentiality of a given event is possible. When observed the event 'solidifies' into the world we know. When enough people see it in the same way the solidity is semi-permanent inasmuch it changes very slowly over time. In this way the world both exists and does not exist when it is unobserved. As an example there is the old question, "If a branch breaks in the forest and there is no one there to hear it, is there any sound?" My answer would be a resounding "No!" It is not until the vibration of the branch breaking hits the mechanism of the ear of the listener that any sound can be heard. It is a matter of perception and interpretation.

The Brain

Thus the brain is a very sophisticated complex chemical/electrical system, installed in and part of a body that experiences the polarity of a dualistic take on things. Although the brain is primarily a reactive system, it's complexity means that it appears to have a separate, solid, permanent, continuous and defined existence and most people live within this system for most of their lives. The brain functions on repetition, habit and the safety of the known with some perceived risk thrown in for window dressing. Cycles of activity are long and numerous enough to keep this fact hidden from most people.

This is consensus thinking when the majority in groups or nations agree to see the same things in the same ways at the same time and anyone who doesn't is mad, bad or different. If they are perceived as intelligent or powerful enough they may be seen as eccentric or artistic. The brain convinces us that we have an individual personality that is also solid, separate, permanent, continuous and defined and has us working to preserve that 'image' of ourselves which really doesn't exist in the limited way we think it does. Hence we seek firm foundations, we repeat familiar behaviour, think reassuring familiar thoughts and seek to 'own' bodies, homes, possessions and experience within rigid time/space concepts. From an open and aware, rather than a perplexed or torpid, perspective, some of this thinking can be quite useful and enable us to live full and productive lives within the dualistic experience.

Consciousness

Consciousness is the focus of our awareness of the moment. It is basically what we are. It is conscious awareness that brain thinking confines, like the pool of light thrown on objects in a dark room, until it is forced to give it up at death.

However, conscious awareness is much more mobile than we are generally led to believe. It is quite possible for consciousness to have a range of non-brain experiences while alive and, at times in everyone's life, non-duality 'sparkles through' (as Ngakchang Rinpoche puts it) to give them unforgettable 'peak moments.' In a paradoxical way, non-duality is sometimes experienced as a 'guardian angel,' 'god,' or 'goddess' which acts as a sort of anthropomorphic bridge which consciousness can cross and re-cross. This is the hidden connection between brain and mind that is sometimes experienced in dreams and meditation.

Mind

Mind is both ours individually and everybody's collectively. It is pure Qi-sense and we usually perceive it and everything within it, in terms of the consensus reality in which we dwell. This is what makes it so confusing as everybody describes it in the same way but slightly differently.

Mind is 'the spirit that entered the land' during the dreamtime of Australian Aboriginal myth. Mind functions at the quantum level. This is at the event level that quantum theory terms 'micro-tuberoles.' These events can occur in more than one place at the same time but are held together by quantum entanglement or coherence. This is known as super positioning in space time geometry and is a fundamental property of the interconnectedness of mind. In terms of what is known as the non-locality theory, mind is spacious, vast, cloudless, choice less, non-dual and penetrates everything including brain. At some level conscious awareness experiences mind but this is blocked or hidden by dualistic thinking. Mind is energetic in nature and part of every level of density and dimension, including time, space, matter and energy and is most importantly non-dual. Non-dual is not the same as whole or oneness. It is none of what the Buddhists

41

call the four philosophical extremes of monism, dualism, nihilism and eternalism. These along with ritualistic ideas belong to dualistic brain thinking. Non-duality must be experienced by conscious awareness and this is possible for everyone. Some people attempt to explain this experience in terms of what is known as 'twilight language' and paradox. The Taoists do this as does the Zen koan and, the Dervish describe it in a rather beautiful way as 'longing for the beloved.' Some modern physicists call this the 'zero point field' and new astronomers describe it tentatively as 'quintessence.'

The energy of mind is like a clear light that is focussed through the brain. The brain separates the light into the five rainbow colours of the elements. However, most brains distort the clear colours of the rainbow and leads conscious awareness to experience dualistic conditioning and conceptually negative forms of thinking and behaviour. What we see hear and feel is a conceptual interpretation of what is happening. What is happening is spacious and perfect. It is our interpretation or concept that is the perplexed experience of dualistic conditioning. This is why the space element or as some term it 'ether,' is not empty. It consists of the resonance of subatomic Qi-sense. The space element is closest to the non-dual nature of mind which is a plenum of unconditioned potentiality, infinitely malleable, moulded or shaped in respect of all five elements by becoming the object of thought. It is the very stuff our world is made of. Thus conscious awareness forms it through the step down of energy into the dualistic world we know and love but is the subject of our continued addiction. Prior to becoming the object of thought it is non-dual, spacious and perfect. It is this perfect, spacious, sky-like state that is the meditative experience.

Thus mental disorder occurs when conscious awareness is completely overwhelmed by brain activity. This may take place to the point where conscious awareness is no longer 'conscious' of what is happening. At this point conscious awareness either retreats into the spaciousness of mind or becomes isolated from both mind and brain. This is the most painful experience we can suffer. However, at some point it is always 'aware' of what is happening, hence the pain. Everybody 'knows' what they are doing all of the time. In this way 'sanity' is the degree to which conscious awareness functions smoothly in relation to both mind and brain. Some people say that this can be measured. So, in the final analysis we must acknowledge that we are in and of the physical world and we must strive to order our existence, both positive and negative, with energetic clarity.

Polarity, mental disorder and the rainbow colours

The unconditioned potentiality of the plenum is distorted in five ways according to our perception of the rainbow colours of the five elements and this is reflected in the degree of perplexity or clarity experienced. Depending on the depth of the distortion of the transparent Qi-sense of mind, the kind of mental disorder experienced will range from mild to severe depending on the degree to which conscious awareness is wise to the self perpetuating nature of distracted brain activity.

The mechanism through which brain limits conscious awareness is based on the distortion of the clear, transparent energy of mind as it passes through the brain and becomes the vibration of the rainbow colours of the elements. The relationship between the degree of each distortion and the relationship of each distortion with the other within the five elements becomes the focus of the move toward clarity. In severe cases the distortion is complete and conscious awareness does not experience clarity at all. This leads people to the notion of evil and the psychopathic personality which presents difficulties in terms of the help that may be offered. But even in these cases transparency does 'sparkle through' on odd occasions. Transparency is the resolving third between perplexity and perfect purity, that reflects a state beyond the here and now and is beyond the scope of this work.

Just as clear, transparent Qi-sense increases in density as it 'steps down' toward what is experienced as matter, the same is true of the finer vibration of what is experienced as thinking. The denser vibration of thinking becomes distorted by brain activity (brain is matter and thus at the same vibrational density as the body), which is primarily expressed through the emotions of joy and love, being themselves examples of transparent expressions and closer to mind, while hatred and fear are examples of perplexed expressions of brain dominance. Mental disorder moves toward the ultimate forms of distortion which fall into definite types which can be mapped through reference to the five elements. Interestingly, these can be seen to match, to a certain extent, modern psychiatric classifications. However, I believe that diagnostic classifications are mostly unhelpful. They give a false sense of knowledge and understanding to the worker and serve only to label and stigmatise the mentally disordered.

Thus the five distorted perceptions may be viewed as ways of coping with consensus reality. Consensus reality can be explained by paraphrasing Descartes, "We think, therefore, I am." It is this conceptualisation of negative emotions through brain activity that causes the problem. Negative emotions and negativity can be expressed with clarity and are not necessarily undesirable. We live in a polaric world and it is the blockages and distortion of energy that need to be cleared and eliminated. In this way mental disorder can be viewed as a normal response to an abnormal perceptual situation. However, open flow of Qi-sense is the natural state of the body/brain complex making all mental disorder a workable situation. The problem can be viewed as healing in action because we are self regulating self healing beings. Even in the worst cases of what psychiatrists would call 'functional or organic psychosis,' there are moments of clarity when the transparent nature of mind sparkles through bypassing the perplexity and distortion of brain activity.

Thus the difference between mental wellbeing and mental disorder is one of degree on a sliding scale. It is the difference between transparency and perplexity. The more conscious awareness is able to perceive the Qi-sense of the mind and the five elemental colours with clarity and transparency the greater the opportunity for a healthy open response to life situations. The more conscious awareness is limited to a perception of distortion and perplexity through repetitive brain activity, the greater the chance of chaotic and difficult reactions to life situations occurring. Mental wellbeing is spacious and aware, mental disorder is dense and blocked. Perception is achieved through the relationship of the rainbow colours of the five elements experienced through the metaphor the five senses expressed as positive and negative emotions and the ever changing balance of the 'divine proportion.'

We will now briefly examine the main elements and their sub modalities that form useful correspondences to the main thrust of working with the five senses in respect of mental disorder.

The colour of the space element or Qi-sense is blue. The space element is related to all five sense perceptions. The 'emotion' is ignorance The perplexed perception of this element is the feeling of being overwhelmed and not understanding who or what you are and your place within the world. Insensitivity and a dull humourless attitude predominates. This equates to the psychiatric classification of psychopathy. The transparent perception is of clarity and unlimited intelligence that is peaceful and contemplative.

The colour of the air element or motility is green. The related sense perception is touch. The perplexed perception is one of panic and seeing menace in everything and everywhere. People expressing this perception are jealous, power hungry and competitive. The emotion is desire. This equates to the psychiatric classification of paranoia, delusions, anxiety and obsession. The transparent experience is one of self accomplishing activity that is confident, practical and positive.

The Modalities of the Elements

Key:- sense – emotion – perplexity – transparency – psychiatric condition - colour

Space – Qi-sense

All senses – ignorance - bewilderment – clarity – psychopathy – blue

Air - Motility

Touch – desire – power hungry – grounded confidence – paranoia – green

Fire - Combustion

Hearing – pride – insecurity – compassion – psychosis - red

Water - Fluidity

Sight – fear – aggression – clarity – depression – white

Earth - Solidity

Taste & smell – greed – dominance – equanimity – personality – yellow disorder

---

The colour of the fire element or combustion is red. The related sense perception is hearing. The perplexed perception is one of obsessively grasping, insecurity, isolation and loneliness. The emotion is pride and the psychiatric classification is psychosis. The transparent perception is of awareness, compassion, passionate communication with everything and total appropriateness in thought and action.

46

Turned on and tuned in!

The colour of the water element or fluidity is white. The related sense perception is sight. The perplexed perception is anger and aggression being self-righteous over analytical and 'picky.' The emotion is fear. The related psychiatric classification is depression. The transparent perception is clarity, integrity, luminosity and intellectual precision.

The colour of the earth element or solidity is yellow. The related sense perceptions are taste and smell. The perplexed perception is fixity and dominance expressed as territoriality being avaricious and arrogant. The emotion is greed and the related psychiatric classification is personality disorder. The transparent perception is equality, equanimity, expansion wealth and generosity.

States of Being		
Perfect Purity	Transparency	Perplexity
This state can be experienced	Being *in* the world and *of* it This state can be lived	This state can be endured

There are essentially three states of being; Perplexity, Transparency and Perfect Purity or non-duality. In this work, we are concentrating on moving from perplexity or mental disorder, that is a state that can be endured, toward Transparency and openness, a state that can be described as living well. Perfect purity contains both Perplexity and Transparency. Perfect purity, or non-duality, is a state that pierces through the other two states. It is a state of being that can be experienced but is beyond the scope of this book.

Over the years I have devised a specific method for working with the polarity of transparency and perplexity through the five elements, the related sense perceptions and emotions and this is the subject of the next chapter.

Here in the fractal garden, there's enough room for our dreams and dark doubts, our discoveries and slow evolution. There's room to grow in, so we needn't be perfect, or failing that, be cast out. Perfection is end-stopped, but this garden allows change. Here we can still walk with divine nature that is visible everywhere, yet finally unknowable. Its majesty stretches beyond our human ken into darkness, yet it willingly shares as much as we can bear to see.

Katya Walter

CHAPTER 3

Toward a Method of Working

"Men will always be mad and those who think they can cure them the maddest of all." Voltaire - 1762

First considerations

This chapter gives the foundation for the more specific techniques outlined in chapter 4. However, we must be very clear at the outset what we mean by 'methods of working.' We are not attempting to 'treat or cure' anyone. The only true healing is self healing. Each person has all the resources they need in order to heal themselves. Thus every individual is responsible for their own healing. The most that we can agree to do is to work with them toward gaining the power to do so—to establish the free flow of Qi-sense—to enable empowerment. A metaphor for this process is of assisting someone stuck in a car in the snow. We could do many things, try to tow them out, call a motoring organisation, give them coffee and sandwiches, go for help etc. But all we really need to do is give them one inch of wheel grip to send them on their way under their own volition.

Ethics & value base

In considering methods of working with people having mental disorder it is important to have a clear understanding of issues around values and ethics. Initially I took the view that it is important to have a clear ethical stance and value base springing from whatever secular or religious system one subscribed to as an individual. However, I have come to the view that a 'clear ethical stance and value base' is a somewhat arrogant and partisan position leading to overt or covert feelings of moral superiority. Secular and religious belief systems spring from fear and are a form of mental enslavement that usually mean the same reaction to a multitude of different situations in which individuals find themselves. Clear open responses require flexibility and often an abandonment of our own position. This is source of fear for many people. Fear of making a wrong or inappropriate response.

This sort of thinking is the very essence of the power relationship. The power relationship has its base in fear. When we engage with someone's pain through our own fear we begin to feel pity and this leads to sympathy. A frightening but powerful position. Someone once said that if you want to know where to find sympathy, it is in the dictionary between shit and syphilis!

When we engage with pain through positive regard both for ourselves and the other person this creates an equality that leads to empathy and thus compassion. The base of our wisdom is our knowledge and theory. The base of our compassion is our action and methods of working. Through wisdom and compassion we lose our worst fear—the fear of making a wrong or inappropriate response that will bring the world down on our heads. The basis of all fear is the fear of death fuelled by loneliness and isolation. Thus we distort the perfection of mind and use the resulting distortion as evidence that we exist as solid, separate, permanent, continuous and defined. It is from this distorted perception that our perplexed thinking and action arises. The transparency of interconnectedness negates this error. Thus we are moving beyond the notion that there is a specific problem causing the disorder which is one step further than looking at symptoms.

Acknowledging the dark side

It is important to acknowledge that we keep the darkest parts of ourselves well hidden under layers of rationalisations. All sentient beings have the capacity to be ruthless, sanguine, brutish, violent and inhuman. At some time in our life we most certainly will, to a greater or lesser degree, all behave in these ways. Most people are ashamed of this capacity within themselves and hide it from themselves through a process of denial. One of the ways in which we justify this behaviour was called by the sociologist David Matza 'techniques of neutralisation,' In which our own behaviour is justified in terms of perceived errant behaviour in the victim. A classic example of this was the National Socialists in Germany blaming the Jewish population for all of the ills befalling the society so that they could persecute them.

Harvard psychologist Stanley Milgram conducted an experiment in learning in which he set out to prove that not only the Germans are capable of the kind of behaviour that took place in concentration camps—we all are. Given the right set of circumstances, belief system or persuasion by authority, we are all capable of the most extreme acts of cruelty and violence. This is something we need to be very aware of in the caring arena because we often have a lot of power over the lives those we are working with.

All cultural bias is a manifestation of this behaviour. It is usually a sophisticated excuse to persecute one another. Humans have a great propensity to dominate and make slaves of one another. This is deeply distorted and perplexed thinking. Acknowledging that we have the capacity to behave in such ways actually mitigates against such behaviour taking place. Moving toward clarity and transparency enables us to side step such behaviour traps which damage the perpetrator as much as the victim.

These behaviours spring from negative emotions and can

be classified as; any kind of bullying, oppression or inappropriate touching, violence (visual, verbal or physical), greed without regard for self or others and sex without positive regard for the self or the other person (although anything consensual is fine). Sadism and masochism are difficult issues. I once spoke to a home help who after the initial visit was refusing to return to the home of a bereaved man. It transpired that he had asked her to whip him as had his wife for the past thirty years, both of them deriving a great deal of pleasure from the practice!

We have strange attitudes in this country toward sex and violence. I can remember a time when it was considered acceptable for wives and children to be severely beaten 'when they deserved it.' It was also a widespread view until recently that child sex abuse just did not happen. Acceptance and denial are still rife. It is estimated that about 160 women a year are killed by their male partners, but I am not aware of seeing the headlines in the papers about this kind of crime once a fortnight. It is also estimated that sexual necrophilia is quite commonplace, the perpetrators doing work, not wanted by many people, in hospitals and mortuaries. However, as I have found on courses, even police officers and social workers do not want to acknowledge or talk about it, and the dead don't complain.

Being aware of these issues and confronting negative emotions with ourselves and others are essential in our work. Clarity and transparency are the watchwords.

Two fundamental needs

For mental wellbeing all people have two fundamental needs. The first of these is to receive positive regard from at least one other person. The second is to do or be involved with something that the individual and at least one other person consider to be worthwhile. Having a relationship with another person is of paramount importance because it frees up the context of the person's life. Being involved with something worthwhile means that the person is accepting responsibility for themselves and their behaviour. This is the root of the empowerment position. A person who is mentally disordered will always lack, or believe they lack, one of the above. They will have no raison d'etre, no reason for being. This will cause pain. fear and negative emotions. Bringing this into the open at the outset is of paramount importance. Becoming involved and agreeing to work with the person may be a way to begin to fulfil these needs – change behaviour and feelings will follow.

Stages of mental disorder

As indicated previously, everybody has all the resources they need in order to heal themselves and live well. All that we can offer to do is work with them when they have decided that healing is necessary. We are in the role of consultant, helping the person to develop their own healing techniques. The body, which includes the brain is a wonderful self regulating system. All that is necessary is to free-up the flow of energy in order to feel well.

However, if the person is not ready or does not want to change then we have nothing to work with. In relation to this it has been my observation that there are definite stages to mental disorder that eventually affects the physical organ of the brain in measurable ways. Sometimes this process is long and drawn out over decades sometimes it occurs much faster. There is mounting evidence that the onset of 'dementia' in the elderly can be spotted in individuals in their teenage years.

Basically people appear to go through the following stages. Mental disorder begins as a normal response to a difficult or abnormal situation. It then progresses to become the usual response to any kind of stress. People will seek to hone this response even going to medical textbooks to build a set of symptoms that are acceptable as a diagnosis, for example 'depression.' This is why the diagnostic process or labelling approach is less than helpful and is often instrumental in creating the disorder. At this stage it becomes part of the personality, eventually taking over the whole identity of the person becoming their normal way of functioning. At this point it will certainly be affecting them physically and physiologically, causing chemical/electrical disturbance within the brain and affecting brain and body tissue.

The problem is that once the mental disorder becomes part of the personality, identity and way of life, people will cling to it and fight to preserve it. Any attempt to change this will be seen as an attack on the self. In the words of the song "they are caught in a moment and can't get out of it!" Thus a person will work both covertly and overtly to protect the disorder so we must be watchful because a person may actively seek help on the basis that, "I tried 'x' therapy and even that did not work although the therapist was wonderful." In the final stages it is almost impossible for the person to work toward health. However we must also be aware that these things will not always be in the open and the person may also be fooling themselves that they wish to become well.

When I first started working with mentally disordered people I believed that they all wanted to become well and would, with help, move toward this position. This was a naive and erroneous belief. We must be aware that some people will have much of themselves invested in the disorder. People engage with their pain because there is a payoff. This payoff may be that they have a secure place of power and prestige and a certain notoriety within the disordered state. They are prescribed expensive medication, have the attention of highly paid medical professionals, are receiving benefit payments, attend support groups with a wide circle of psychiatric friends and do not have to go to work on a daily basis while having a topic of endless discussion and interest.

In this way I believe that everybody knows what they are doing all of the time, even the most 'psychotic' individuals. I remember in the early days of my practice spending many hours on the wards with diagnosed schizophrenics who would stand on one leg in a strange attitude for hours on end and were thought to live in their own world unaware of what went on around them. However, after long hours, when I did manage to communicate with them, it became apparent they were acutely aware of what was happening, shift patterns, who was on duty, the names of their children, who was sleeping with whom etc, In the case of those suffering from depressive stupor who were thought to be totally uncommunicative I also found, given enough time, these people were well able to discuss and understand their situation. This is useful knowledge because we know that however disordered the person, anything said in their presence is likely to be understood. Therefore however hopeless the situation may appear there is always the possibility of movement and change. This way of working can be very time consuming and it is much easier to offer an hour long consultation and prescribe drugs which mask the symptoms that make us uncomfortable.

Unless it can be accurately assessed that a person wishes to seek wellbeing it is impossible to begin working with them. We are working with wellbeing not repeat business! First, we must discard the payoff then the healing must involve collaboration at a very deep level.

Working toward clarity & transparency

We are attempting to move toward what the ancients called gnosis and I term 'transparency,' the knowledge and understanding of our own condition and our relationship with the world we perceive. The role of the worker in this is to some extent to act as a mirror and attempt to give the person an experience of what it feels like to have gnosis/ transparency. In this way it is important for the worker to have a personal experience of transparency. Thus they must personally be practitioners of the methods they advocate. As I have already hinted, the bottom line is that the worker must be involved. They may be the one offering the unconditional positive regard. The one who finds something the mentally disordered person does as being worthwhile.

Working from a perspective of clarity there is no room in this relationship for petty convention or morality or the encouragement of this or that course of action. In this way we do not suggest that people give up conventional treatment. We move them toward a position of constant questioning and open examination of all the issues from their own unique perspective and away from passive acceptance. We are seeking to foster response rather than reaction. Thus if they are told to take a certain drug they will require a detailed explanation of its effect and side effects, the outcome if the drug is not taken. They can then make an informed decision. This is empowerment. Of course the difficulty here is that they might not do what you think they should.

Finally, some people hold that we are all suffering from mental disorder. I hinted at this earlier writing of the 'depth' of distortion reflected in the degree of transparency or perplexity experienced. Thus I would define mental disorder as the inability to respond in an open and healthy way to life situations. It is all repetitive reaction. Most of us experience degrees of transparency and perplexity that are dependent on any number of variables. However, at all times our method here is to work toward transparent response rather than perplexed reaction. Hence the ideas of working with mental disorder presented here may be viewed at many different levels across a spectrum from 'normal' to 'psychotic.'

How does the brain work?

Although the brain is just a basic chemical/electrical system, in function it is extremely complex and it is this that enables it to lead conscious awareness away from transparency and into perplexity. Most models of the brain view it as a kind of computer with the ability to record what happens to us in our lives. A sort of on/off binary device functioning through neurotransmitter systems. However, the brain can also be viewed in another way that is more useful to an empowerment model of interaction.

At the moment, the language we use to discuss the brain comes from computation and this is inconsistent with what we know about the brain. It positively does not store and order information and construct images by processing rows of digits in a binary fashion like a microchip. We know that the brain is composed of arrays of neurons that act like maps and represent the entire cognitive and sensory qualities of events and objects.

Thus memory is not a stored picture gallery. Remembering, in fact all cognitive functions, involve interactions between maps in many different areas of the brain and a reconstruction of the most likely item needing to be displayed. This fits with the most recent quantum thinking which suggests that events and objects exist as limitless potentiality and it is observation that 'congeals' them into the events and objects we perceive.

It is now thought that the brain is more akin to an analogue processor, dealing in whole concepts and their relationships to one another. It does not deal in bits and pieces of data. This means it functions effectively not by using hard data in a linear fashion but through analogy and metaphor. This has real implications when working with mental disorder where the tools of analogy and metaphor are often of more use than rationality.

The three approaches

In promoting mental health the key word is empowerment. We work as a consultant advisor to the mentally disordered person. To enable an understanding toward working practices, it is helpful to use two sets of three connected distinctions that indicate disturbance in distinct areas of human functioning and the causes of this disturbance.

It is useful to consider working with cognition, body and expression, through thinking, behaviour and affect. Of course, this distinction is made for convenience, to enable us to work toward empowerment with the person within the confines of consensus reality. Cognition, body and expression are really different densities of Qi-sense.

The causes of these disturbances in the three areas of human functioning arise from physical considerations, levels of vulnerability and events that cause stress. Most people are able to cope with quite high levels of physical difficulty and discomfort, with feeling vulnerable and stressed at various times during their lives. It is when they all occur at the same time, or together in very high levels, that the person may be overwhelmed by mental disorder. The level at which mental disorder may occur will differ from individual to individual but these events will be present in every case of perplexity or what Breggin terms 'overwhelm.'

These approaches inform the specific techniques outlined in the next chapter when we look at working with the energy of the mental (cognitive), physical (body) and emotional (expression) being.

Working with the five senses

Everybody experiencing mental disorder will have, in a greater or lesser degree some disruption of the senses. This is inevitable because the senses are our only way of interacting with the here and now. Our five 'outer senses' are complimented by five 'inner senses' and to a great extent we only ever experience things in our heads and hearts, what in the east is called the 'heart-mind.' Thus the five senses are the vehicle by which we represent what we perceive as our outer environment to our inner world. We access our outer senses through physical exercise and our inner senses through relaxation meditation and trance. A blending of the two working in harmony gives us transparency.

The modalities of the five element system give us a way into working with mental disorder through the five senses. We process our thoughts and experiences of the world and interact with other people solely through our five senses. Some people have posited a sixth sense. I believe it is useful to view this sixth sense as a combination of all the senses in the way that the whole is greater than the sum of its parts. In fact all the methods and techniques in this book are directed toward the development of multi-sensory awareness. Using our five senses in concert leads to a balanced resonance of our being between our internal and external worlds which is one of the facets of transparency. Of course poor use or denial of one or more of our senses or perhaps over use of one or more sense at the expense of the others, inevitably leads to perplexity.

The five senses can be classified as visual, auditory, kinaesthetic, olfactory and gustatory or sight, sound, touch, smell and taste. We use these senses to create a sort of personal interactive map of the world. We attempt to keep some parts of the map static while we allow other parts to change according to our reaction or response. Our ability to change and adapt our map while remaining centred in the here and now reflects our degree of transparency. On the other hand rigid definitions and unchanging features are signs of perplexity and fear.

The discipline of neuro-linguistic programming explores

these themes in some detail and provides some very useful insights. NLP holds that the olfactory and gustatory systems are composed of remembered smells and tastes and are mainly concerned with the primal urges of survival such as food and sex. It is interesting that these are the primary ways in which people ingest mind altering drugs, breathing them in or swallowing them as food. The visual, auditory and kinaesthetic senses are the prime senses we use to interact with other people and the world and knowledge of a persons preferred use of these different senses can aid communication.

Visual: people who are visualising will hold a posture with their head up or level and their neck muscles are likely to be contracted. They will breathe high in the chest and their voice will be fast and higher pitched. Their eyes will look up or be defocused. Corresponds to light.

Auditory: auditory thinkers tend to make small rhythmic movements of the body often swaying from side to side. The voice tonality will be clear and expressive, often musical. They will hold their head to one side (telephone position) and their breathing will be in the mid range. Their eyes will be midline looking to the left or right. Corresponds to sound.

Kinaesthetic: kinaesthetic thinking will involve a head down, rounded or slumped posture. The breathing will be low in the abdomen and the voice tonality low and soft, even dreamy. The eyes will look straight down maybe glancing right or if internal dialogue is also involved glancing down to the left. Corresponds to touch.

We generally use our senses in some kind of medley or individually depending on the situation. However, everyone will have a dominant mode and using the appropriate phrases for the appropriate sense will aid communication. Please refer to the chart for the eye accessing cues and phrase examples.

Predicates and Eye Accessing Cues

Some examples are given below of linguistic predicates and eye accessing cues that may indicate the types of thinking processes that the speaker is using. By matching these predicates you can build rapport and gather more information from the speaker.

Predicates

Eye Accessing Cues

Visual

Remembered images   Constructed images

I *see* what you mean...
I get the *picture...*
We need to *focus* on this aspect..
This is how things *look.....*
Thing are *looking* up.....
Show me what you mean.....

Auditory

Constructed sounds   Remembered sounds

I like the *sound* of that.....
I *hear* what you are saying...
He *told* me everything....
Let's get into the *rhythm* of this....
This is a *harmonious* way of working....

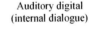

Kinaesthetic

Kinesthetic
(Feelings and bodily sensations)

Auditory digital
(internal dialogue)

I like the *feel* of that...
I *sense* what you mean...
You must be under *pressure...*
She's very *hot* on these issues....
Lets get things *moving......*

Working in the here and now

Perhaps the most powerful tool we have is working in the here and now. In life the only thing we ever have to cope or deal with is that which is happening right at this very minute, now! We must practice accepting the here and now as if it had been chosen: this is the way to empower yourself. Always work with what is in front of you as the Tibetan Dorje Trollo says, "as it is, may it be like that, as it happens, may it happen that way, there is no purpose attached to events." Therefore, always work with the moment, don't try to resist it or control it—go with the flow as the hippies used to say. It will change your life beyond recognition.

When I attend the dentist, I have no numbing injections. Not even for root fillings. This is a cause of much discussion at the surgery. I laugh it off by saying, "where there is no sense, there is no feeling." The answer, however, lies in accepting the here and now. Many years ago when working in a therapeutic setting, I was very keen on this idea and did a lot of study and practical work through meditation and martial arts training. I also practised at the dentist. Whenever there was pain, I just went with it, no resistance, no grasping, just acceptance. As if like magic, the pain stopped and I have never felt it since. I was in the zone, the meditation space. I had experienced the valuable lesson of 'being' in the 'here and now.'

In actual fact it is not possible for anything to happen outside the here and now. When we believe that it is possible, we suffer all sorts of pain and negative emotions as a result. When events occurred in what we call the past it was actually the here and now. When events occur in what we call the future it will be the here and now. Understanding this at the level of direct experience will lead to transparency—and perhaps pain free dentistry.

Achieving transparency

The sole aim of the methodology, methods and techniques in this book is to move from a surfeit of perplexity and achieve a greater degree of transparency. This does not mean that perplexity goes away it just means that our perception of it is different. This is the paradox of life, that things can only be known in relation to their opposites. Perplexity is also known as distraction and torpor and a host of psychiatric diagnosis. A good illustration of perplexity is those times when we know all the words but just can't seem to get the tune. Although most of us are deeply perplexed and need to move toward transparency, this does not mean extinguishing perplexity. Perplexity is a necessary catalyst to our experience of this place we call the world.

Transparency is a state known by other names such as congruency, openness, clarity and spaciousness. It is 'wu wei' – doing without action. It leads to a balancing of the five senses, (inner and outer) and means being centred, comfortable and joyful. It is a focussed state in which our whole being runs in one direction. It is total relaxed attention to what we are doing in the here and now. A position where the five senses, thought, language and behaviour all compliment one another and move simultaneously in the same way. The picture we make has no clashing colours and the band are all playing the same tune. Transparency is an 'empowered' rather than a 'powerful' state. It is when we realise with all our hearts that we are solely responsible for our reaction or response to the flow of events in our lives.

Sky Blue

Meditation is adventure
the greatest adventure
the human mind can undertake. Meditation is
just to be
not doing anything – no action,
no thought, no emotion.

You just are and it is a sheer delight. From
where does this delight come when you are not
doing anything? It comes from nowhere,
or it comes from everywhere.

It is uncaused because the existence is of the
stuff called Joy.

Osho

CHAPTER 4

Specific Working Techniques

"What these scientists have discovered is nothing less than astonishing. At our basic level we are not a chemical reaction but an energetic charge."
Lynne McTaggart

The techniques outlined below are simple and very powerful ways of working with our bodies and the intrinsic Qi-sense. If approached carefully and incrementally they have no poisonous side effects, but do require the sort of commitment where they become part of the person's way of thinking, doing and feeling. These basic techniques start the process of movement away from perplexity toward transparency. They require planning and effort on a daily basis. Success is not a once only thing, it is an everyday, everyway thing! The worker should carry out the procedures alongside the person with the mental disorder. There is a saying in Polarity Therapy "give a treatment and you get a treatment." We are all on the curve, we are just at different places. These procedures are a starter pack which will be effective if practised daily, or at least on a regular basis. However, please refer to the further reading section for more specific and detailed additional material, available in books. on video and via the internet.

Purpose of techniques

In any case of mental disorder it is always best to start work from the physical aspects of being, focusing on the body/brain responses through the five senses. The purpose of the techniques outlined is to stimulate and balance the

Qi-sense of the person undertaking them, toward transparency. Body and brain are part of the same system, get the resonance moving and the stagnated body and brain will follow, allowing conscious awareness to experience transparency. At all times we are really working with different densities and degrees of wobble, stagnation or blockage of the intrinsic resonance of Qi-sense within the here and now.

In this chapter, the metaphor of the five energies will be merged with the modalities of the five senses as a way to work with the cause of mental disorder. Primarily, we will be working with the useful duality of exercise and meditation seeking 'stillness in action and action in stillness,' toward the triunity of a balanced expression of transparency. This is a moving living harmony of activity. purpose and fulfilment through an open and sky like interface of conscious awareness with our five senses. We seek to achieve the sparkling free flow of the resonance of intrinsic Qi-sense in our relationships with each other and the here and now of the world in which we find ourselves. What we are attempting to do with these techniques is to achieve multi-sensory awareness.

Music

Music is a very important enhancer of the auditory representational system and so we start working with our sense of sound.

The ancients were very well aware of the effect that musical vibration had on the human organism. It is emerging in modern scholarship just how much of our mystical and scientific thinking has come almost undiluted from the ancient Egyptian civilization via the Greeks and Romans. In ancient Egypt physicians were always priest or priestesses of the lioness headed goddess Sekhmet. These celebrants would study the chants for some twenty years in order to become 'Makheron' and could sing a perfect wave form of sound each time they chose to aid their own spiritual practices and to undertake healing. Some modern writers suggest that the great pyramid is a huge sounding box centred on the king's chamber and that chanting within the chamber either healed or gave psycho-spiritual experiences to any person lying in the stone sarcophagus in the centre of the chamber. This would certainly fit with Pythagorean teaching about the nature and organisation of the vibration we call sound. Some modern practitioners are able to produce this perfect wave sound and we are now in a position to measure this electronically. It has been suggested they are able to heal bones shattered beyond repair by passing this perfect vibration through their hands to the afflicted part and thus reorganise things at the Qi-sense level. Certainly, research has been undertaken and duplicated with musical compositions such as Mozart's piano concerto no 23 – K488 and the music of the Greek folk singer Yanni. Among volunteers diagnosed as suffering from dementia it was found that performance improved in complex tasks like paper folding after listening to such music. It was also found to reduce the number of seizures in people with epilepsy. Rats were also found to negotiate a maze faster after listening to K488.

It is suggested that the music must be well organised and emotionally consistent. It should exhibit long term periodicity, that is, the forms are repeated regularly but not very close together. This mirrors human behaviour and thinking and resonates with brain function. Thus I would suggest that when carrying out any of the techniques highlighted there should be a background of such music.

The above is very useful when disorder is present and we are moving away from perplexity toward transparency. However, in terms of creativity and flow, the rigid confinement of the bar line structure is of little help. Eastern music with its different rhythmic structure and mixing of meters returns to a more natural flow that corresponds with

71

the flow of Qi-sense resonances.

Food

You are what you eat! The second sense we consider is taste, a sense that relies on the third sense, smell. The 'food rainbow' is a balanced mixture of food from the five elemental colours. Red (including purple), blue (including black), yellow (including orange & brown), green and white (32 different shades). In this way our foods are colour coded for our nutritional convenience. Attractive brightly coloured foods tend to be richer in key substances that protect us against disease. Using the visual representational system, ensure that foods from as many different colours as possible are consumed every day. Smell is the other important sense that is used to complement taste. People with colds or sinus problems will often report that their food is tasteless. For a breakdown of the foods into their colours see the diagram opposite. Modern research indicates that there are also five tastes salt, sweet, sour and bitter plus the elusive fifth taste termed 'umami' by modern researchers. Umami is thought to be present in all the other tastes and is a combination of them all manifesting as somewhat savoury. It is supposed to be the taste of 'Almas' the most exclusive and rare caviar in the world—but this could be a marketing ploy. Try it and see!

Smell

Smell is important inasmuch that it aids remembrance of a situation and helps you to naturally get into a receptive state for practice. Many people like to burn incense but I believe that, like smoking, this interferes with the Qi-sense resonance in practice situations. I recommend that you purchase a small burner powered by a candle or electricity that enables the use of essential oils mixed with water to achieve the desired aroma. This is much gentler and less harsh than smoke in a room. If you are able to set aside a room for practice then you

---

The Food Rainbow

Our food is colour coded for our selection convenience!
Primary senses used sight, smell, taste

Blue (Inc. black) Space	Blueberries, blackberries, elderberries plums, blackcurrants, aubergines, black grapes
White (32 different shades) Water	Fish & fowl, bananas, melons, bread, rice, pasta, flour, potatoes
Red (inc. purple) Fire	Tomatoes, strawberries, red meat, cranberries, beetroot, cherries, red cabbage, red onions, red peppers, red grapes
Green Air	Green leaf vegetables and salad, broccoli, Brussels sprouts, wheatgrass, green, peppers, apples, green grapes
Yellow (inc. orange & brown) Earth	Corn, yellow peppers, turmeric, mustard, lemons, grapefruit, wheat, brown bread & flour, oranges, saffron

**this list is not exhaustive.
Attractive brightly coloured foods tend to be richer in key substances that nourish us and protect against illness. Ensure that foods of each of the colours are consumed daily.

---

can build a permanent fragrance within this space that will immediately aid practice.

Compared with our sense of taste our sense of smell is incredibly complex. Received wisdom says that we recognise smells by the shape of their molecules. However, more recent enquiry posits the idea that our noses act like a spectroscope and identify smells by their vibrations or energy signature, so that we are actually aware of what something will smell like long before we actually smell the smell of the perfume or frying bacon. We are thus bathed in a sea of potential smells. Working with our Qi-sense should therefore connect us with ever more subtle fragrances which can be used to identify our mental and physical states. Externally stimulating and internally arousing the memory of smells can be used to bring about desired characteristics within our physical and mental being.

Posture

In terms of the sense of feeling the importance of posture is vastly underrated. Posture is the same as stance in Yoga and Karate. You will have noticed that people with mental disorder undergo distinct postural changes. In some cases the head is lowered the eyes down, shoulders drooped and a shuffling gait. In other cases the head is held back and jaw line thrust forward and they appear tense 'ready to leap' with quick jerky movements. Even in our ordinary everyday lives we sit and stand in abnormal positions in relation to both work and relaxation. This upsets the body balance and blocks the flow of our Qi-sense. Psychotic individuals often stand in extremely odd poses for long periods of time. I believe this is a misguided attempt at self healing. They are trying to realign the body and establish the free flow of Qi-sense. The body does have a perfect alignment and we must attempt to experience and re-establish this, if only for short periods of time. This is the basis of structural balancing. For all the exercises outlined below wear loose comfortable clothing

Basically we must lift the head to raise the spirit, lower the shoulders to sink the elbows, curve the back to soften the chest, loosen the waist, co-ordinate the top and bottom halves of the body and check weight distribution. Be aware that in the west we think in our brains and chest and that this can leads to anxiety and rush. Begin to learn to 'sink your thinking from the head and chest to the heart and abdomen.' This will affect your view of the world and make you more balanced and grounded.

Perfect Posture or Wu Ji

The standing 'empty' posture of balance and stillness is known as the 'Wu Ji' Whether standing, lying down (relaxation) or sitting (meditation and trance), the fundamental body alignments will be the same as this Wu Ji posture. (see the illustration on the next page)

Procedure: stand with your feet shoulder width apart, like the base of a pyramid with your toes parallel and facing forward. You should feel your weight sinking and extending into the ground. Feel your toes relaxing and spreading apart.

Your knees should be just 'off lock' allowing your forward facing hips and lower abdomen to relax and sink somewhat as if you are about to sit down. Let your shoulders drop, 'a release of all tension' allowing your chest to rest in a natural position, not puffed-up nor pulled-in. Allow your consciousness to move from your head and upper chest, where it has been held by tension, to the heart and abdomen.

This enables the spine to be erect but curve naturally.

Your arms should be hanging loosely with a nice natural inward curve toward your body. Make sure the fingers spread and curve.

*Your eyes should look directly forward in a relaxed fashion. You may close them if you can maintain your balance. Feel your head as if suspended by a silver cord from the fontanel. A **very slight** lift should occur **slightly** lengthening the spine.*

This posture should deepen and ease your breathing. It should gently fill your whole lung capacity without being forced.

This posture is very important so work with it, experiment until you get the ideal stance. Remember there is an inside and an outside awareness here.

Standing & moving exercises

I learned five standing exercises from a Japanese martial arts instructor more than thirty years ago. I used them to good effect for fitness and as an alternative to sitting meditation. In fact, during some sitting meditation the resonance was so strong that I had an urge to stand up. During the 1980's I followed a television series 'Stand Still and be Fit' by Lam Kam Chuen. This Chinese 'Sifu' raised the standing exercises to an art form which he called Zhan Zhuang (pron. Jam Jong) and this significantly deepened and widened my own practice. Without a doubt these exercises have an impact on the resonance of our Qi-sense.

The benefits of these standing exercises must not be understated. They are apparently simple—you need to pay attention to detail—but are incredibly powerful. There are five basic positions that correspond to the five elements and thus the five senses. The first posture is the wu ji already described and illustrated opposite. I suggest you start your practice with this posture, standing initially for 30 secs, morning and evening. and building up to five minutes. When you are comfortable with 5 mins, begin doing the posture on one leg, raising the legs alternately to about knee level and pointing the toes back toward the body. Start with 1 min building up to three on each leg. Have a clock with a second hand in view so that you can time yourself. When you are comfortable with this consult Lam Kam Chuen's book and video, for further practice.

There are three points, or Dantian, on the body that correspond to the three representational systems already mentioned. The first is the fontanel at the top of the head; related to light and sight. The second is located in the belly at the point of the golden section of the body, related to sound or vibration and is known in Japan as the 'Hara' and by the Dervish 'Kath.' The third is located on the soles of each

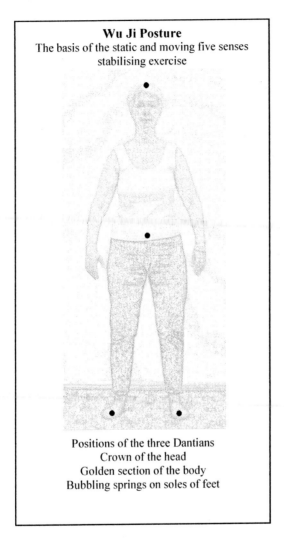

Wu Ji Posture
The basis of the static and moving five senses
stabilising exercise

Positions of the three Dantians
Crown of the head
Golden section of the body
Bubbling springs on soles of feet

foot; relating to feeling or groundedness and are known as the 'bubbling springs.'

I have indicated the positions of the 'three Dantians,' that correspond to the three representational systems, on the Wu Ji diagram above. It is the basic posture for the standing and moving exercises. While practising this standing exercise it is helpful to imagine being suspended by a silver thread from the fontanel which lifts you very slightly to extend the spine. At the same time imagine a vibrating silver/grey pearl of energy at the Dantian that is slowly expanding during practice. Lastly, imagine the bubbling springs on the soles of each foot extending into the ground and anchoring you powerfully but gently. See the paragraph on trance for indications on how to go about this kind of 'imagining.' You should feel for any subtle changes in the body or mental attitude that occur while standing in wu ji.

There are five element moving exercises that compliment the static exercises but you will need to see these demonstrated. I suggest you purchase the book and video by Morag Campbell listed in the further reading. The video also includes another practice called the 'Eight Brocades' which form the basis of martial applications.

Relaxation, Meditation, Trance

For each of our external senses we have a corresponding inner sense and it is these that we engage in relaxation, meditation and trance. Our inner world is limitless. It can represent everything in our outer world, however huge, with ease and still have plenty of room to spare! The primary sense used here is sight or perhaps more properly 'insight.' The other senses are engaged in a supporting role. For instance we might chant mantra or vaporise essential oils. It is interesting to note that chanting mantra silently within the heart/mind engages the same physiological processes as if we had actually heard the sound out loud. This is useful for those who might feel stupid or embarrassed using their voice in this way.

Relaxation: the relaxation response is not meditation, but it is the starting point. Being relaxed you might be peacefully aware or just fall asleep, especially if you relax lying down. During relaxation you can simply mull over your problems or

78

Relaxation Exercise

First start your music! You may sit or lie for this exercise. Close your eyes. Breathe evenly and use the full capacity of the lungs without effort. Make sure the spine and skeleton are correctly aligned and that there is no constriction of internal organs. Start by just letting the body go. Be aware of the muscles and just let the tension flow out of them. There should be no effort here, it should be very natural, very nice, pleasant and non-specific.

Now start to concentrate on specific parts of the body. Start with the top of the head and ears, feel them softening, think of the skin on the face like a blanket over the bones becoming smoother, softer. Now the back of the neck and the spine, the large sets of muscles either side of the spine, relax, relax. The throat, feel the air slipping into the lungs unimpeded. Now the chest and stomach. Feel the lower abdomen rising and falling gently with each breath. Now go down each arm feel the fingers give a little twitch as the tension runs out of the ends. Now feel the muscles relaxing in each leg and feel each of the toes as the last of the tension runs out of the end of each of them. Now let the mind relax and the cares of the day flow away into the distance.

You may fall asleep at this point, but that's okay—you will wake up refreshed. You may stay awake but feel very comfortable—as if you could stay there forever—that's fine too.

just daydream. Cultivating the relaxation response is the first step toward valuing the physical body—an essential for wellbeing. It is through working with and changing behaviour, that feelings follow. It is behaviour over time that leads to physical difficulties and mental disorder. As some writers have put it 'your biography is your biology.'

Meditation is all of the above and more! Meditation is a technical thing and not exclusively a spiritual practice. However, once the technique has been learned it can be used for a variety of purposes including spiritual development and self healing. You do not 'empty your mind' – this is simply not possible. However, you can experience 'emptiness' which again is both a technical and a spiritual thing that will be explained later.

Some writers suggest that meditation was first discovered by early hunters—this is called the hunting paradigm. In order to hunt successfully it is suggested that early hunters would have to sit in cover waiting for their prey. They had to remain relaxed and still but ready to leap at the appropriate moment. They had to keep their minds active and in the moment. This 'relaxed but alert' state is just what is needed to meditate. It evokes a mental pattern called the 'alpha state' a measurable condition during which the frequency of brain waves is reduced. Researchers believe that children spend significantly more time operating in the alpha state than adults and that this enables them to adjust to new ideas and learn faster. We tend to lose the ability as we get older so it is necessary to re-learn it, but, like riding a bicycle, once done it is never completely forgotten. Paradoxically, you can gain more control over wandering thoughts by paying attention to them than by trying to ignore them. Meditation is working with the brain. The brain is part of the body. Meditation is sometimes known as 'silent sitting.'

Basically there are three ways of sitting that have been used traditionally. Firstly, there is what I call the 'Egyptian posture,' that is, sitting in a straight backed chair with the hands palms down flat on the thigh of the same side. The upper body should be as for wu ji posture making sure that the spine is erect but curved and not touching the back of the chair. The seat should be slightly padded so that you are not distracted by discomfort. The feet should be shoulder width apart flat on the floor. It is important to make sure the seat is of the right height so that the knees bend at a comfortable right angle. Pad the seat or put something under the feet to adjust as necessary. You may also fold the hands loosely in the lap lightly resting the right in the left, palms upwards. This is the posture I recommend and that I find most people prefer. This is also the way the 'future' (who some say is already with us) Buddha Maitriya is portrayed meditating.

The second posture is sometimes known as the 'thunderbolt posture' and is the one used in Japanese martial

---

Meditation Exercise

Decide how long you wish to meditate and have way of knowing when this time has passed. As a start I suggest that you begin with five minutes and work up to twenty, over a period of one month. Music as desired.

Settle into your chosen meditation posture. At this point your attention will begin to wander—don't worry about this it is normal—just note that it has happened. Start to concentrate on your breathing. It should be easy, through your nose, and go down into your abdomen making your belly rise and fall slightly, then gently out through the mouth. Watch the breath as the abdomen rises and begin to count the breaths with each exhalation. Continue with this throughout the meditation. Your thoughts will begin to wander, what shall I have for lunch? Must remember to go shopping! Don't worry about this, just note that it has happened and return to counting the breaths. At some point you will be able to observe the stream of thoughts in a detached way while concentrating on the breathing.

*Eventually even the recollection of breathing will subside and you will find yourself totally relaxed and alert in the here and now. You will be aware of your parade of thoughts and what is going on around you **but it will not take you with it**—you will not be swept along, but at a calm still centre. It is important **not to try to achieve this state** but just to focus on the breathing and **let it arise naturally**. Be patient it will come! When it does you can stay as long as you want and your outlook on everyday life will be different.*

---

arts for meditation. This is a kneeling posture with the knees together and you 'sit' on the inner edges of the heels. The upper body is the same as for wu ji and the hands are placed palms down flat on the thighs.

The third posture has several variations and is basically a cross legged posture. The easy posture is the same one we all sat in at assembly at infant school. The perfect posture and the lotus posture you can find clearly described in any elementary book on Yoga. Unless you are already comfortable sitting like this, I have found attempting to do so in the early stages of meditation mitigates against success.

Meditation is not knowledge, it is knowing. Knowledge is of the brain, knowing is of the mind. It is important to understand the difference between knowledge and knowing: knowledge is never of the present it is always of the past, when we have knowledge about something it has already happened. Knowing is always immediate and is to do with the here and now. It is impossible to say anything about it, you can only experience it through meditation. An example of this is the word 'strawberry' the name of a certain fruit. You can read about this fruit. its description, size, colour, shape. how to grow it, how to eat it and perhaps its mystical significance. However, this cannot compare with going into a field, seeing the red among the green leaves, the feel and sound as you pluck it from the plant and the wonderful smell and taste as you raise it to your lips and eat the luscious fruit.

Trance: Trance may seem so odd, so way out, even 'New Age.' However, we all experience trance every night when we go to sleep, so it is actually quite a normal part of our lives. Most of us experience very little during sleep although many people remember dreams which can be quite perplexing. It is possible to retain consciousness through sleep and practice what is called lucid dreaming but that is beyond the scope of this book.

The kind of trance that we will be working with is a

Trance Exercise

Having achieved your meditation state, close your eyes and become aware of your inner self as the focus. Now take a journey back and enter the womb at the point of your actual conception. Pause for a moment and start to move forward through time, through your growth as an embryo and the drama of your birth and then on slowly through all the stages of your life to the present time.

As you do so imagine you are trailing a silver cord behind you that starts with the moment of your birth where you tie a knot in it to acknowledge that fact. Proceeding through your life the cord extends with you becoming longer and longer. Pass through all your life experiences, pausing here and there to register happy, sad or meaningful events, some loss or new awareness, each time recording them by making a knot in your silver cord. When you reach the present you should see your silver cord with its event knots trailing behind you. Pull it toward you so that you can tie the babyhood end to the present end and lay it on the ground in a circle in front of you. Now step inside.

Depending on your temperament you may now like to imagine that you are sinking down into the earth or rising up in the sky, perfectly safe and comfortable within the silver cord of your circle of life. At some point, different for everyone you will reach your inner or outer limit and effortlessly begin the return journey to your starting point

As you reach this point, you become aware that in front of you will be what some people call the inner pilot and others call the Spiritual guide. They will give you something that is your unique symbol to access them in the future. This symbol can be anything from a flower to a cross. You have accessed the divine aspect of yourself for learning, further travels, help and guidance.

---

waking trance that follows and builds upon the relaxation and meditation experience. It is sometimes called 'guided mediation' among other things. There is a language of trance.

We all remember at school when the teacher told a story it would begin "Once upon a time..." or "If you're sitting comfortably I'll begin..." Watch what happens when these words are spoken to any group of people, they immediately shift a physical and mental gear. There is an air of expectancy. We can develop our own trance language which once in our meditation space will launch us into many unique experiences. On the previous page, as a starter, and from numerous possibilities, I give one example of a practice based on the Lion People exercise given by Murray Hope.

This sort of work can give us the divine experience which aids toward healing. The opposite is divine illness from which we get the word 'devil.' Another kind of trance that comes unasked is epilepsy and some kinds of temporal lobe epilepsy can give the person an experience of union with a Godhead or other divine beings. Pythagoras said that in terms of thinking and meditation we must be like the best of charioteers. This metaphor works on many levels. Basically if the charioteer lost presence for even a moment disaster would ensue, not for them drifting off into dualistic mind stories rooted in past and future.

Walking

Walking is quite simply the best exercise there is. It takes us back to the developments that are said to have taken place during our hunter gatherer lifestyle and are still with us. Even the clockwork view of thinking holds that exercise increases serotonin levels and aids neurotransmitter activity.

The great advantage of walking is that it can be done anywhere. It is better when there is peace, quiet and little traffic and on grass or earth surfaces rather than tarmac or concrete. There are even machines that allow you to walk in the comfort of your conservatory or living room.

To be useful it should be done over measured distances

and include different speeds and levels of incline, getting a little breathless with light sweating at least once during the walk. In order to do this you need to measure your pace and time yourself over a certain distance. Once you know the length of your pace you can measure distances by counting them. Going on regular walks with landmarks at specific distances is the best way to approach this exercise.

Example of an Intensive four week starter walking programme

Week 1. Walk on level ground 200 – 600 yds at a speed of 2 – 3 mins per 100 yds for the first two days. Take a 2 min break every 100 yds. Days 3 and 4 take a break at each 200 yds. Days 5,6 and 7 go without stopping.

Week 2. Walk on level ground 400 – 800 yds at a speed of 1 – 2 mins per 100 yds for the first two days. Take a 2 min break every 100 yds. Days 3 and 4 take a 2 min break at each 200 yds. Days 5,6 and 7 go without stopping.

Week 3. Walk on level ground 800 – 1000 yds, complete the whole distance in 20 mins. Days 1,2,3, and 4 rest as you wish. Days 5, 6 and 7 rest for 5 mins half way.

Week 4. Walk on level ground 2000 yds, have 5 min rest half way. Complete each half in 20 mins

- Always time your walk and know the distance walked. This gives a sense of achievement.
- Try to walk with another person or form a group.
- Attempt to walk on 'softer' surfaces like grass or a firm sandy beach where possible to avoid wear and tear on the joints.
- Circular walks, or out one way, back another, are best because you avoid the feeling of repetition.
- Build up a repertoire of walks and write them down in a note book. Keep a diary of events, feelings and people you met during your walks. Note the changing seasons etc.

Timing yourself between landmarks then becomes easy with an inexpensive watch or pedometer from a discount store or a very expensive chronometer from a sports shop! Walking should ideally be done every day. It is good to experience the seasons and note the changing year. It is also helpful to experience the vagaries of nature as long as you don't get a chill.

Reprise

What we are attempting to achieve with these techniques is multi-sensory awareness that will move us toward a transparent existence within ourselves (inner senses) and the world (outer senses). As we become more experienced at multi-sensory awareness we begin to notice that we only ever experience anything, however solid it may appear, through our interpretation of sensory input. This input, despite our belief to the contrary, is constantly changing and is therefore essentially impermanent. At this point in our practice and meditation we may have the experience of the emptiness of all phenomena. It is with this experience that the real work begins toward an appreciation of non-duality. Our most important assets in this process are our sense of joy and sparkling good humour. As one of my correspondents signed off recently, 'love and twinkles!'

Life is lived

Death is not lived, though its coming may be experienced.

Scott Shaw

CHAPTER 5

Beyond the Fear of Death.

"The origin of all fear is the fear of pain and death" Anon.

This chapter could change your death!

It has been said many times and in many places that the only real fear and the one from which all other stem. is the fear of death. Certainly I have found this to be a preoccupation among mentally disordered people. I believe that in this society we have a very unhealthy attitude toward death. We don't want to read or talk about it and usually our only experience are the versions we see in war or crime films where we are at once removed and at the same time know to be pretend. It is for this reason that on the spot news reporting that shows death on television, leaves us unmoved because we have seen representations of it as drama. Unfortunately, we still have the nagging remembrance that it will eventually happen to us and our loved ones that ultimately manifests itself as our fears displaced onto other things. We know that brain thinking is very good at leading us astray in just this way. However, the only thing that makes any system of thought valid is our own belief in that system. Knowledge and understanding can change belief. Metaphor can also give us insight in this way and lead to 'knowing'. Thus the Dervish refer to death as their wedding—their wedding with eternity!

Elemental dying

The Philosopher Pythagoras (circa 6[th]C BC) established a mystic school on a hill overlooking the town of Croton in southern Italy. Over the gate the legend *Eskato Bebeloi* - 'no entry for the profane,' was inscribed and although entry to the school and Temple of the Muses was extremely difficult, in a situation unusual in ancient times, men and women were admitted on equal merit. There were as many enlightened Pythagorean women as there were men.

It is said that the Pythagoreans chose the time of their death. They would retire to the Temple of the Muses and having given up food and drink would sit quietly waiting for death. They apparently had a technique for collapsing the elements of their bodies into themselves through the energy centres or what are now commonly known as the 'chakras.' This was evidenced by vivid colours surrounding their bodies during this process. culminating in a beautiful light turquoise blue as the consciousness returned to the non duality of the mind through an opening in the top of the head. It is said that at this time the physical body had disappeared completely and it is for this reason there are no verified tombs for Pythagoras or any of his community.

A fanciful ancient story we might think. However, in modern times I have met people who claim to have witnessed similar events among Dzogchen practitioners in the Himalayas. These people usually retire alone to a tent or cave to take 'rainbow body' which is a direct result of their spiritual practices that include exercises to physically open the skull bones at the fontanel to allow the mind essence to leave the body. This rainbow of colours is said to be a result of the elements collapsing into themselves in a specific order and the colours that are seen by viewers of this phenomena are the five colours associated with the elements red, white, blue, yellow and green. In this case, however, the body does not disappear completely as the hair and nails remain to be placed in reliquaries as objects of veneration. This may be cultural.

So is there any truth underlying these reports? Is there a process or order associated with dying which is the same for all of us but has been missed or ignored by modern scholarship? In the past I have supervised and assessed staff in nursing homes where the experience of death is a daily occurrence. It would be my contention that it is possible to observe elemental dying in ordinary people although in these cases we are still left with the disposal of the physical body!

Stages of the dying process

Drawing on Pythagorean and Dzogchen ideas and my own personal observations the following process appears to be apparent. Although each death is unique according to the circumstances, the physical condition and the state of mind of the dying person, a general process can be identified which always takes place either slowly or quickly depending whether the death occurs through sickness or old age or through accident or violence. Obviously the former via the deathbed experience is more easily observed.

In the first stage, the dying person experiences the dissolution of the earth element through the base energy centre or chakra as it dissolves into the water element. The person is overcome by drowsiness and dullness and feels heavy and pressed down. The senses of smell and taste disappear, the head lolls, the teeth grind and the body seems to shrink. There will be a yellowish hue about the person.

In the second stage, the dissolution of the water element takes place through the navel chakra as it dissolves into the fire element. The person suffers extreme dryness of mouth nose and throat as blood and bodily fluids coagulate. Bodily sensations are greatly reduced, the sight blurs and the person becomes irritable and uncomfortable. The skin and hair seem to lose their lustre and the yellow haze seems to change to smoky white.

In the third stage, the dissolution of the fire element takes place from the heart chakra as it dissolves into the air element.

It becomes impossible to swallow and the heat leaves the limbs and moves in toward the centre of the body. The sense of hearing fades and the exhaled breath becomes colder. It is at this point that the person ceases to recognise even close friends and relatives The smoky whiteness surrounding the person starts to show blotches of spreading redness.

The fourth stage brings the dissolution of the air element through the throat chakra as it dissolves into the space element. The person will begin to hallucinate and there is a rasping in the back of the throat, the so called death rattle, the person loses the sense of touch and a green hue will be visible. At the fifth stage the entire energy system and polarity of the body collapses into the sky like dimension of the space element and leaves the body through the top of the head at the fontanel. This centering of polarity through the space element is sometimes described as the essential white drop of energy received from the father at conception, which is located in the crown chakra moving down through the central channel to the heart chakra. At the same time the essential red drop of energy, received from the mother at conception, rises from the base chakra to the heart chakra. As the drops merge the moment of death is over and all aspects of consciousness melt into the spaciousness of pure mind. At this point the pure spacious non-dual mind rises and leaves through the crown of the head. It is at this point that a faint, clear bluish hue may be noticed. Of course we are not actually viewing 'something' 'going somewhere' but merely a shift of conscious awareness. It is all 'refined energy,' 'Dao' or 'the zero point field.'

It is not necessary to be clairvoyant to witness the rainbow colours of the dissolution of the elements. Caution is obviously needed at the deathbed due to the primitive way in which death is viewed, especially in this country. However, one can point out the mistiness around the body that is always present during the dying process. This may be due to the condensation of bodily fluids or perhaps reasons related to the energy of the person. However. most people can see this quite clearly. Ask the person to imagine what colour the mist is and they will generally see the appropriate elemental colour and are then able to observe the whole process.

The above is a useful and powerful thing for us to know and experience. This does not mean that the fear will leave us just by reading about what happens. Work is required. Work on ourselves and with others.

Start from where you are

We must begin this work with knowledge and understanding. Brain thinking is compulsive and addictive and leads ultimately to complete perplexity. It tries to prove that it exists as a permanent, unchanging state, but this is false because it is transient and changing. It is this fear, the fear of losing itself, of death, that is the real problem. The fear of death is fuelled by loneliness and separation. This is the paradox of the striving for permanence through consensus reality and the terror of separation from it leading to fear. The world reflects what we hold in our heart/mind. A violent person full of anger and fear will have a vastly different experience to a loving, transparent person who seeks to know and understand.

The concept of death is dependent on the notion of the time/space continuum rooted in consensus reality. In actual fact there is no reality, only perception. Time and space are conceptual abstractions. Each one of us perceives a completely different world that we place in time and space. We agree to come to a consensus about what we see and this is what we call reality placed in time and space. Starting soon after our birth we spend our whole childhood and early life learning what this consensus reality is about and how to function within what is effectively a perceptual prison. By the time we are adults we believe it to be a true and only representation of the world. The system is not totally rigid and there is some room for flexibility, however, go too far and you are deemed mad. Past, present and future are the props of the semi-rigid flexibility and allow it to appear to change over time.

In actual fact everything takes place in an ever present here and now. Our limited perception cannot cope with everything happening at the same time so it separates events into past, present and future within space—the space/time continuum. We use our perception to focus on events within this manufactured continuum like the beam of a torch in a dark room. Our perception is actually very limited and deletes, distorts and generalizes our experiences to make them manageable within the field of the continuum.

Thus time is really a conceptual abstraction and it is only at the moment of individual experience that the illusion is strong enough to hold as if it is real. At all other times it is viewed as the multifaceted event that it really is when viewed by many people. In the popular imagination time runs in a line and some people even acknowledge that there can be many different time lines for the same sets of events. However, they are caught in the linear trap. It is thought that if we go back along a particular time line and change even one event catastrophe will ensue in the present within that time line, perhaps with people disappearing forever. If we 'went back in time and changed things' the only thing that would change would be our perception of our particular focused view of the now. The myriad of other slightly different perceptions would remain the same and consensus reality would not be affected. Even if every perception changed greatly it would only be the perceptions that changed and not the event that is a perceptive illusion. Events reflect the interplay of the resonance of Qi-sense and our bodies and brains are part of that interplay. In actual fact, consensus reality is malleable and changeable but we all adjust our perception to cope with this happening.

Sometimes, some of us can't cope with believing the assumption that it is real. So we throw off the conditioning leading to problems which can include mental disorder but may be viewed in other ways such as brilliance and genius. This will certainly include the suspicion that we don't really exist in the way we think we do.

Loss of personality

Thus we live in fear of death because we are seduced by brain thinking and consensus reality into believing we are something we are not. We believe in a personal, unique identity. However, upon examination it is discovered that this identity relies on all sorts of props, our name, our life story that exists in the past, dreams of the future, family, home, job etc. Take them all away and what is left? This world can be very convincing until it is removed by death and we no longer have these places to hide. Death is just the loss of another social role.

Our personality changes slowly but constantly all through our lives but very quickly at the moment of death as all the elements that support it collapse into one another and finally into spaciousness. We are actually never the same person from moment to moment. We all believe in a personal, unique and separate identity but this is merely a mask a reference point to fend off impermanence and escape the cosmic paradox in which everything exists by contrasts.

Through meditation we can begin an alert witnessing of all the roles of the personality. By experiencing the Qi-sense resonance as your reference point you are empowered to see through the control dramas of brain thinking and its servant the personality. We are thus able to move from a position of transparency toward timelessness, naturalness and perfect purity that are beyond the fear of death.

Once you have experienced the 'emptiness' (Sunyata) of

all phenomena life and death are never the same again!

Blue dye comes from the indigo plant, But is bluer!

Ice comes from water, But is colder!

from; Xunzi Quan Xue

One interpretation of these verses:

'The student must exceed the teacher. Be more than you are.'

Appendix 1

Psychotropic Drugs

It has been recorded since the beginning of history (and probably before) that people from all over the world and in all walks of life have ingested substances that change the physical and mental quality of their lives for a variety of purposes from religion to recreation. As was discovered during prohibition in the USA and world-wide since that time, no amount of law making will prevent people using psychoactive substances.

Although it can be said that the purpose of all drugs is to reduce pain, this is accomplished through the desire to bring about four main states:

- the wish to relax or chill out
- the wish to wake up or get energised
- the wish to change or improve mood
- the wish to experience expanded consciousness or get connected

It is possible to achieve these states by taking psychotropic drugs, especially if it is carefully managed. If taken regularly the effects are short term. anything from six months to two years depending on the individual. Unfortunately, no drug is 'target specific,' (although some people will tell you they are), and they impact on virtually every system within the body/brain complex. Eventually, the system largely comes to terms with them and they cease to have the desired effect and become part of normal functioning, this is usually called addiction, at which time to stop taking them will have dire consequences, unless done slowly over a period of time.

In modern times the supply and regulation of drugs is the province of government, the pharmaceutical industry and 'freelance suppliers.' The problem with freelance suppliers and street drugs is that they are almost always impure, being mixed with other, sometimes vastly toxic, substances in order to bulk them out and increase profits. It is also virtually impossible to obtain reliable measured doses and strengths. Even the drugs licensed by government, like alcohol and tobacco, are adulterated with harmful substances by manufacturers for a variety of reasons. This invariably leads to pain, sickness and even death. sometimes over long periods of time.

The main supplier of psychotropic medication is 'Big Pharma,' the world-wide multi-national, multi-billion dollar drugs industry. Psychopharmacological substances are designed and produced in huge laboratories, the same basic set of drugs being brought out by different companies in slightly different formulations under brand names. New types of drugs are being constantly sought and hailed as the new cure all. Prozac was an example of one of these.

These psychotropic medications are universally prescribed to people suffering from mental disorder. They all have undesirable side effects, varying in degree according to the constitution of the individual taking them. Drugs appear to provide a very expensive chemical straightjacket that subdues human emotion, feeling and creative urge. On the plus side they will be administered in an unadulterated form and in measured doses, however, these can be extremely high. There is also a widespread reporting back system in respect of side effects. In the case of side effects being noted other drugs will be developed or prescribed to counteract them, with still more to counteract the side effects of those drugs and so on ad infinitum. I have known patients on fourteen different drugs, only one of which was prescribed for the actual disorder, from which the person was still suffering symptoms. It has been my experience that the amount of ignorance about psychotropic drugs among the general medical profession is staggering. Specialists will be offered large research grants and all sorts of gifts such as lavishly produced books, expensive pens, mugs, post-it notes and of course free samples of the drugs, to positively examine the effects of particular drugs thus ensuring that it is prescribed.

Within the medical and allied professions psychiatric medication is seen as more helpful than harmful and in some cases a universal panacea. Having heard thirty-five years of testimony from those who have taken the drugs and those who have prescribed them, it would be my view that they are at best useless and at worst extremely harmful. Some people would argue that they actually create mental dysfunction. Certainly drugs advocates would take the view that it is not the drug that leads to adverse effects and behaviour but the 'illness.' In the arena of mental disorder this is a very difficult thing to disprove. Certainly, it is clear from observation that in the early stages these drugs do impair higher mental functions, especially creativity, and mitigate for any number of unwanted side effects. Some writers would also argue that the therapeutic level of dosage is the same as the toxic level of dosage.

Unfortunately, non-medical professionals and alternative practitioners feel obliged in most cases to refer their clients for medical evaluation in the case of mental disorder. This will almost certainly lead to the prescription of medication. Sometimes this occurs on the first visit to the medical practitioner and the patient is told they will probably have to take it for the rest of their lives!

I believe that therapeutic models, educational, social and spiritual, including the ideas in this book, are far more effective than drugs in encouraging and empowering people with mental disorder to come to terms with their problems and live more fulfilling lives of perfectly pure, spacious transparency.

Appendix 2

Perfectly pure, spacious transparency is all there is...

The world we see is our sensory interpretation of a fluctuating field of Qi-sense. (This Qi-field is mind and created us to observe itself—but that's another story) This Qi-field responds to being observed by our conscious awareness and is interpreted through our brain. This is why the Buddhists say that the world is exactly as it should be; nam jang – perfectly pure. It is only the brain's interpretation of it that cause ripples, blockages and difficulty. Christians might call this Qi-field God. If we take charge of our thinking as Christ and Buddha did. We will view the Qi-field as it is—nam jang!

Each time we see the same object or event this is the brain's reinterpretation of the Qi-sense—thus we never truly see the same thing twice. In this way we do not see the same object but a similar interpretation that usually conforms to consensus reality. Consensus reality means that people in similar groupings tend to interpret the Qi-sense and see things in the same way. Thus all humans will see a similar world in large. However, different groups will see objects and events differently according to socialization, belief etc. These groups are on a scale from millions strong to individuals holding their own interpretation. Thus everything is the same but everything is different.

Mental disorder sometimes means that the interpretation of the Qi-field is vastly different from general consensus reality. This is however, also a matter of interpretation because, as an example, the religious fanatic might seem mad to some but holy to others. The disordered view of consensus reality is really just a different interpretation of the Qi-field which is why some people who are disordered enough for the rest of us not to make sense of what they are saying can often understand one another's view of the world.

As an example, consensus reality is why people tend to see the same images in terms of ghosts and aliens. The black robed hooded monk in lonely places is a case in point. In pre Christian times he might have been viewed as a Shaman dressed in a dark blue robe with a broad brimmed hat pulled down over one eye. As the consensus reality changed so did our interpretation of the Qi-sense. In fact a viewing of this figure can be induced in test subjects through mild electrical stimulus of certain areas of the brain. Temporal lobe epilepsy can also produce incredible spiritual experiences which some people liken to being one with God. These are in fact the brain reinterpreting the Qi-field.

The Qi-field is present at all 'times.' In fact, it only ever exists in the here and now. Brains separate this here and now into past, present and future as another interpretation of the Qi-field because the brain cannot cope with the perception of everything happening at the same time. At the quantum level every possible event is available constantly and this one of the reasons why in some cases people are able to view events from the history of a place as if in apparition. It is just a previous consensus reality impressed on the Qi-sense and retrieved by the brain. In the unconditioned Qi-field the potentiality exists for all events and objects to take place—it just needs to be perceived in that way and this is why great thinkers appear to change the world. But at the end of the day it's all perception, interpretation, lack of clarity and thus illusion. Don't get caught up in it—nam jang is all there truly is...

All worldly pursuits have one unavoidable
and inevitable end, which is sorrow.
Gains end in loss
Buildings in decay
Attachments in separation
Births in deaths...

Milarepa - Tibetan practitioner and poet

Knowing this we are thrown back upon the
present, on this moment, right here, right now,
for that is all there truly is...

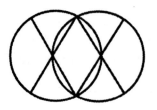 Regeneration

Trust what you do
And just do it

Antonia Walter

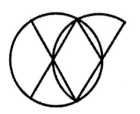 Degeneration

Suggested further reading & viewing list

*Peter Breggin - Toxic Psychiatry – Flamingo

ISBN 000637803X

Morag Campbell–Quinta-Essentia–Masterworks International

ISBN 0954445007 & Video 'Chi-Kung, Series 1.'

*Ngakpa Chogyam 8 Khandro Dechen – Roaring Silence
Shambhala ISBN 1570629447

*Lam Kam Chuen   The Way of Energy - Gaia

ISBN 1856750205 & Video 'Stand Still 8 Be Fit.'

Joel Kramer 8 Diana Alstad – The Guru Papers – Frog

ISBN 1883319005

Lynne McTaggart - The Field – Harper

ISBN 0722537646

Joseph O'Connor & Ian McDermott - NLP –Thorsons

ISBN 0007110375

Michael Scneider – A Beginner's Guide to Constructing the Universe - Harper

ISBN 0060169397

*Eckhart Tolle - The Power of Now Hodder/Stoughton

ISBN 0340733500

Katya Walter – Tao of Chaos - Element

ISBN 1852308060

*indicates other relevant works have been written by this author. Most also have excellent websites.

Contact details for books and videos in respect of standing
and moving exercises

Morag Campbell
Masterworks International
27 Old Gloucester Street
London WCIN 3XX
0780 3173272
Moving exercises – Book Quinta – Essentia
Video: Chi Kung series 1

Lam Kam Cheung
The Lam Association
1 Hercules Road
London SE1 7DP
020 7261 9049
Standing exercises – Book: The Way of Energy
Video: Stand still and be fit

Coming in 2004

By Tony Caves

The Art of Mental Wellbeing
Stillness and Motion—the Workbook

Printed in the United Kingdom
by Lightning Source UK Ltd.
99862UKS00001B/211-213